The Art of Clinical Practice in Optometry

FRANK EPERJESI
HANNAH E BARTLETT
MARK C DUNNE

Copyright © 2020 Frank Eperjesi
All rights reserved
ISBN: 9798642979631

DEDICATION

To everyone who wants to get better.

CONTENTS

DEDICATION i
FIGURES v
PREFACE vi
ACKNOWLEDGMENTS vii
ABBREVIATIONS viii
SECTION 1 PRE-REFRACTION 1
Chapter 1 History and symptoms 2
Chapter 2 Measurement of visual acuity 14
Chapter 3 Focimetry of a cylindrical lens 25
Chapter 4 Brückner test 27
Chapter 5 Hirschberg corneal reflexes 29
Chapter 6 Assessment of pupil function 30
Chapter 7 Cover test at distance 34
Chapter 8 Cover test at near 40
Chapter 9 Prism cover test 41
Chapter 10 Near point of convergence 43
Chapter 11 Accommodative amplitude 45
Chapter 12 Random dot stereograms 47
Chapter 13 Oculomotility 50
Chapter 14 Cover test with oculomotility in nine positions of gaze 55
Chapter 15 Interpupillary distance 57
Chapter 16 Trial frame set up 59
SECTION 2 REFRACTION 61
Chapter 17 Spot retinoscopy 62
Chapter 18 Near fixation retinoscopy (Mohindra technique) 65
Chapter 19 Jackson cross cylinder (JCC) 67
Chapter 20 Binocular balancing 70
Chapter 21 Binocular addition 72
Chapter 22 Determination of the near addition 73
SECTION 3 POST REFRACTION 77
Chapter 23 Maddox rod 78

Chapter 24 Maddox wing 83
Chapter 25 Distance and near Mallett Unit 87
Chapter 26 Direct ophthalmoscopy-anterior segment examination 93
Chapter 27 Direct ophthalmoscopy-posterior segment examination 95
Chapter 28 External and anterior eye examination using direct illumination   97
SECTION 4 FURTHER INVESTIGATION 99
Chapter 29 Pulsair™ non-contact tonometer calibration 101
Chapter 30 Pulsair™ non-contact tonometer procedure 102
Chapter 31 Goldmann tonometer calibration 104
Chapter 32 Perkins tonometer calibration 105
Chapter 33 Drug instillation 106
Chapter 34 Perkins and Goldmann tonometer procedure 107
Chapter 35 Visual field analysis patient set up 110
Chapter 36 Goldmann perimetry 112
Chapter 37 Humphrey visual field analyser 117
Chapter 38 Gross perimetry-confrontation and peripheral fields 121
Chapter 39 Henson Pro visual field analyser 123
Chapter 40 Ishihara colour vision test 132
Chapter 41 City University colour vision test 133
Chapter 42 Amsler grid 134
Chapter 43 Pelli-Robson contrast threshold chart 137
Chapter 44 Modified monocular indirect ophthalmoscopy 139
Chapter 45 Head mounted indirect ophthalmoscopy 141
Chapter 46 Slit lamp biomicroscopy 144
Chapter 47 Slit-lamp ophthalmoscopy with negative lenses 147
Chapter 48 Diagnostic contact lens and gonioscopy 151
Chapter 49 Examination of the anterior chamber 154
Chapter 50 Examination of the iris 158
Chapter 51 Examination of the vitreous 159
SECTION 6 SPECIALIST BINOCULAR VISION 161
Chapter 52 Monocular estimate method (MEM) dynamic retinoscopy. 162
Chapter 53 Low neutral dynamic retinoscopy 163
Chapter 54 Accommodative facility 164
Chapter 55 Vergence facility 166

Chapter 56 Detection of ARC using the Mallett Unit 168
Chapter 57 Bagolini lenses 170
Chapter 58 Determination of the AC/A ratio 173
Chapter 59 Eccentric fixation 175
Chapter 60 Jump convergence 177
Chapter 61 Prism cover test 178
Chapter 62 Fusional reserves 180
SECTION 7 CONTACT LENSES 183
Chapter 63 One position keratometer 184
Chapter 64 Two position keratometer 186
Chapter 65 Upper lid eversion 188
Chapter 66 Slit-lamp calibration using patient's eye and general set up 190
Chapter 67 External and anterior eye examination using direct illumination 192
Chapter 68 Corneal examination using direct illumination 194
Chapter 69 Corneal examination using indirect and retroillumination .. 197
Chapter 70 Corneal examination using specular reflection 200
Chapter 71 Fluorescein staining 201
Chapter 72 Using a Wratten 12 barrier filter 204
Chapter 73 Tear meniscus evaluation 205
Chapter 74 Soft contact lens insertion 207
Chapter 75 Soft contact lens fit assessment 208
Chapter 76 Soft contact lens removal 210
Chapter 77 Gas permeable lens insertion 211
Chapter 78 Gas permeable lens fit assessment 212
Chapter 79 Gas permeable lens removal 214
GLOSSARY 215
AUTHOR BIOGRAPHIES 225
INDEX 227

FIGURES

Figure 1 Example history and symptoms recording 13
Figure 2 Brückner test-R reflex brighter. 28
Figure 3 Brückner test- equally bright reflexes R and L. 28
Figure 4 Cover test eye movements in right esotropia. 35
Figure 5 Cover test movements: alternating esotropia with left eye preference. 36
Figure 6 Checking for a heterophoria when conducting cover-uncover test. 36
Figure 7 Checking for a heterophoria when conducting cover-uncover test. 37
Figure 8 RAF rule with vertical line target for measuring NPC 43
Figure 9 TNO stereopsis test. 47
Figure 10 Cardinal positions of gaze. 50
Figure 11 Duction movements of the right eye. 53
Figure 12 Classification of version movements. 53
Figure 13 Maddox rod: red line seen by patient when grooves are vertical. 79
Figure 14 Add appropriate prisms to left eye until line passes through the spot. 80
Figure 15 Repeat with MR grooves vertical to test for vertical phoria. 80
Figure 16 Detecting and measuring cyclophoria. 81
Figure 17 Measuring horizontal phoria with the Maddox wing. 84
Figure 18 Measuring vertical phoria with the Maddox wing. 85
Figure 19 Measuring cyclophoria with the Maddox wing. 85
Figure 20 Detecting horizontal fixation disparity with the distance Mallett Unit. 89
Figure 21 Detecting horizontal fixation disparity with the near Mallett Unit. 89
Figure 22 Types of horizontal fixation disparity (same for the near Mallett Unit). ... 90
Figure 23 Types of vertical fixation disparity (same for the near Mallett Unit). 90
Figure 24 Types of torsional fixation disparity (same for the near Mallett Unit). 91
Figure 25 Perkins contact tonometer. 105
Figure 26 Kinetic perimetry and the hill of vision. 112
Figure 27 Blind spot and pathological peripheral field defect left eye. 115
Figure 28 Blind spot and pathological peripheral field defects right eye. 116
Figure 29 Threshold estimation for the Humphrey visual field analyser. 117
Figure 30 Humphrey plot depicting a normal visual field for the RE. 119
Figure 31 Humphrey plot depicting an inferior visual field defect in the LE 120
Figure 32 right eye superior quadrantopia. 130
Figure 33 left eye superior quadrantopia. 131
Figure 34 Metamorphopsia detected using the Amsler grid 136
Figure 35 Central scotoma detected using the Amsler grid 136
Figure 36 Pelli-Robson contrast threshold chart. 137
Figure 37 Recording findings with a single Bagolini lens: right esotropia. 171
Figure 38 Recording findings with a single Bagolini lens: alternating esotropia 172
Figure 39 Magnitude and direction of eccentric fixation 176
Figure 40 Bausch and Lomb (one-position) mires 184
Figure 41 Javal-Schiötz (two-position) mires 186
Figure 42 Zeiss mires 186
Figure 43 Optic section through a healthy cornea. 196
Figure 44 Corneal abnormality illuminated with indirect illumination. 197

PREFACE

Our principal aim in putting this book together was to provide a low cost for novices in the field of optometry that is comprehensive and easy to access and is easy to purchase.

Standard teaching on optometry degree programmes usually involves initially delivering information via a lecture to a large audience using combinations of text-based slides and still images with an occasional short video. This is often accompanied with a paper-based handout and a few key references to be read later. These large group lecture sessions are usually backed up with some small group practical classes which often take the form of a tutorial followed by an expert standard demonstration by an experienced clinician, and the opportunity to practice on fellow novices. Skills are developed and improved through a process of observed trial and error with almost instant feedback from the teaching clinician.

Over the years students regularly asked us for more time to practice clinical optometric procedures especially in the lead-up to formal practical assessments. Because of limits imposed by time and money and the availability of equipment and space these practical sessions usually last between one and two hours on a once or twice weekly basis. In between sessions the students only have still images and text from their class notes or textbooks to which to refer. It is mainly because of these requests from our students that we have assembled this collection of procedures. Videos that assist in understanding many elements of the content of this book are available through subscription from our friends at EyeTools https://eyetools.vhx.tv/.

We realise that the contents of this book and the videos are no substitute for actual hands-on practice with equipment and patients, but we believe that they will be useful resources that can be consulted before and/or after each practical class.

In each chapter we have given a brief introduction, explained the use and then described the procedure. We have also included hints and tips gleaned from our personal experiences obtained during teaching and clinical practice. This is followed by examples of how to record findings, and where appropriate, typical findings.

We hope this book will be useful to those embarking on a career in optometry and those who have been away for a while and those that want to improve their clinical skills.

ACKNOWLEDGMENTS

FE thanks Mark Slocombe Founder Director of Creation Video and Co-Founder Director of EyeTools for his expert assistance in preparing the images. We all three thank those students who have pestered us over the years with their questions. Without them this book wouldn't exist and our work would have been much duller.

ABBREVIATIONS

Av.	Average
GAT	Goldman Applanation Tonometry
IOP	Intra-ocular pressure
LED	Light-emitting diode
NCT	Non-contact tonometry
RE (R)	Right eye
LE (L)	Light eye
VA	Visual acuity
CHP	Compensatory head posture
NMD	No movement detected
Δ	Prism dioptres
PD	Pupillary distance
SOP	Esophoria
XOP	Exophoria
Ortho.	Orthophoria
XOT	Exotropia
RhyperT	Right hypertropia
Alt XOT	Alternating exotropia
Tropia	Heterotropia
Phoria	Heterophoria
DS	Dioptres of sphere
DC	Dioptres of cyl
Ret	Retinoscopy or retinoscope
JCC	Jackson cross cyl
FD	Fixation disparity
LogMAR	Log of minimum angle of resolution
LH	Lea Hyvärinen

SECTION 1 PRE-REFRACTION

Chapter 1.0 History and symptoms

Chapter 2 Measurement of visual acuity

Chapter 3 Focimetry of a cylindrical lens

Chapter 4 Brückner test

Chapter 5 Hirschberg corneal reflexes

Chapter 6 Assessment of pupil function

Chapter 7 Cover test at distance

Chapter 8 Cover test at near

Chapter 9 Prism cover test

Chapter 10-Near point of convergence

Chapter 11 Accommodative amplitude

Chapter 12 Random dot stereograms

Chapter 13 Oculomotility

Chapter 14 Cover test with oculomotility in nine positions of gaze

Chapter 15 Interpupillary distance

Chapter 16 Trial frame set up

Chapter 1 History and symptoms

Introduction
In the medical world it is frequently stated that 70% of diagnoses be made by taking an accurate history and symptoms. This is usually the first and most important procedure in an eye examination and should include questions on:

- General information
- Reason for visit
- Symptoms
- Ocular history
- General health
- Family ocular history
- Family medical history
- Occupation, hobbies and driving.

The main reason for attendance for a patient will determine to a large extent the tests used during the examination. It is imperative that the main reason for the visit is determined and that this concern is addressed in the final summary at the end of the examination.

When examining children, and particularly for those who seem nervous, we find it best to start by conversing with the parent or carer to determine the main reason for the visit. If the child is co-operative from the outset then, once a few preliminary greetings are over, the child can be addressed directly. It is important to discover in the child's own words whether he/she is having any vision or eye problems and if so what they are. We advocate noting the exact words the child uses to describe any visual problems. Sometimes information is obtained in this way that even the carer is unaware of. It is wise to corroborate all statements from children with a parent or carer to check for accuracy where possible. Birth details, illnesses when the child was younger and family history questions will have to be asked directly of the carer.

General information
During the history and symptoms general observations of the patient can be made:

- Overall physical appearance, mobility.
- Thin, twitchy – overactive thyroid.
- Overweight, ruddy faced – systemic hypertension.
- Compensatory head posture (CHP) – ocular motility anomaly.
- Facial asymmetry – congenital anomalies.
- Eyelids – lesions, ptosis, epiphora, entropion, ectropion.

- Eyes – lesions, red eye, nystagmus, strabismus.
- Speech, intelligence, emotional state – choice of tests.
- Age, gender and race – influence the prevalence of some ocular disorders.

Remember to record the date of the examination.

Reason for visit

The response to this question will establish the chief complaint and during the examination the practitioner should attend to this complaint along with all others. This is often referred to as using a problem-oriented approach. Reason (s) for the visit may include a general (routine) eye examination, change in vision or visual acuity, headaches or diplopia.

The reason for the visit allows the practitioner to:

- Consider a list of tentative diagnoses.
- Ask more questions aimed at differential diagnosis.
- Start by asking an open-ended question: Do you have any problems with your vision?
- Obtain a full description of the problem(s).

We suggest use of the LOFTSEA system.

LOFTSEA
Location/laterality
If the chief complaint is headache, ask: Where does it hurt?
If chief complaint is blurred vision, ask: Are both eyes affected?
If chief complaint is diplopia, ask: Does this happen when you are looking in any particular direction?

LOFTSEA
Onset
Ask: When did this start happening?
Ask: Did it occur suddenly or gradually?
Sudden onset may indicate pathology
Gradual onset may indicate that:
Patient thinks that glasses are needed but does not want them.
Problem is not having a severe effect on patient.

LOFTSEA
Frequency and occurrence
Ask: How often does this happen? And: How long does it last?
If problem is of visual origin then symptoms tend to occur:
When using eyes (reading, watching TV, driving).
Weekdays more than weekends.
Start in the middle of the day and gradually get worse.

LOFTSEA
Type and severity
If the chief complaint is headache ask: Is it a throbbing, sharp or dull headache?
If the chief complaint is blurred vision, ask: 'Is the blur constant or intermittent? And: Was the vision loss partial or total?
If chief complaint is diplopia, ask: Is the double vision one-on-top-of-the-other, side-by-side or somewhere in between? And: Does the double vision disappear when one eye is closed?'

LOFTSEA
Self-treatment and its effectiveness
Ask: Does anything make it go away? And: How well does this work?
A patient with asthenopia may stop or reduce the time spent reading.
A patient may take aspirin or other headache remedies.
The problem is more likely to be minor if the patient has done nothing about it.

LOFTSEA
Effect on patient
Ask: Does this affect how well you can do certain things? And: Have you been to see your doctor about this?
The response to these questions may dictate patient management:
A child who has difficulty seeing the board at school is likely to benefit from having distance glasses.
A presbyope who has difficulty reading music may require an intermediate add.
Cataracts that are causing difficulties with daily activities may prompt referral.

LOFTSEA
Associated or secondary symptoms
Ask: Are you having any other difficulties?
These may be associated with the chief complaint, such as, frontal headache caused by squinting to see in the distance when the chief complaint is blurred vision.
Secondary symptoms may not be associated with chief complaint, such as, 'floaters' noticed in a presbyope whose chief complaint is blurred vision when reading.

Symptoms
Some symptoms may already have emerged through the reason for visit. All patients should be asked about:

- Distance and near vision
- Asthenopia
- Headaches
- Pain or burning

- Diplopia
- In high myopes, listen out for symptoms of flashes and floaters.

All symptoms should be followed up using the LOFTSEA technique.

Distance and near vision
Try to ask questions that suit the patient's age and activities of daily living.

For distance vision, ask:

Do you have any problems reading the board?
Is everything clear on the TV?
Can you see road signs clearly when you drive?
For near vision, ask:
Any problems with reading school books?
Can you read the newspaper easily? What about telephone numbers or details on medicine bottles?
Can you see the computer screen clearly?
Constant distance blur:
Myopia – gradual onset (10 and 18 years old), headache (squinting).
Nuclear sclerosis – myopic prescription shift in older patients.
Intermittent distance vision blur:
Young diabetics, variable myopia.
Pseudomyopes, after long periods of close work.
Intermittent near vision blur:
Presbyopes, near vision often okay in daylight or good lighting.
Distance and near vision and blur:
Astigmatism
Pathology – cataract, maculopathy.

Asthenopia
Ask: Do you get any eyestrain?
Asthenopia has many causes:
Listening to symptoms can help differentiate visual causes (see LOFTSEA) from pathology.
Visual causes include – ametropia (most often hyperopia), accommodative dysfunction, presbyopia, binocular anomaly, poor illumination.
Pathological causes include ocular inflammation and retinal disease.

Headaches
Ask: Do you get any headaches?
If yes, follow-up even if patient says headache not caused by vision.
Vision related headaches tend to be:
Associated with use of eyes (see LOFTSEA).
Mild/moderate, dull, non-throbbing.
Located above or behind the eyes, occasionally occipital or temporal.

Pain or burning
Ask: Do you get any discomfort in your eyes, such as pain or burning?
If yes, commonly a sign of dry eye syndrome.
May be to tear anomalies.
May be side effect of medication for hypertension.
May be associated with arthritis.
Patients may complain that eyes feel watery; pseudo-epiphora, reflex tearing caused by dry eye.
May be due to other ocular inflammatory conditions.

Diplopia
Ask: Do you ever see double?
Note that many patients report double vision when they mean blurred vision.
Confirm by asking: Do you see two of everything or does everything seem blurred?
If diplopia, ask: Does the double vision disappear when one eye is closed?
If yes, then binocular diplopia and there must be a binocular anomaly.
Ask: Is the double vision one-on-top-of-the-other, side-by-side or in between?
Pathological/traumatic diplopia more often vertical diplopia.
If no, then monocular diplopia, cataract or irregular astigmatism.

Flashes and floaters
Floaters are common and arise due to normal age-related changes to the vitreous (it liquefies and shrinks).
Flashes (photopsia) are more serious and occur when liquefaction causes posterior vitreous detachment leading to the risk of retinal detachment; this risk increases in high myopia. On eye movement the vitreous impacts the retina causing the photoreceptors to be activated and flashes to be visualized.
In high myopes, it is wise to listen out for reports of increasing floaters or flashes.

Ocular history
Present refractive correction:

- Spectacles
- Contact lenses
- Low vision aids.
- Previous eye treatment:
- Injuries, infections, surgery, treatment
- Last eye examination.

Present refractive correction-spectacles
If unsure, ask: Do you wear spectacles?
If yes ask:

At what age did you start wearing spectacles?
How many pairs do you have?
For each pair owned, identify the type (single vision, bifocals or varifocals) and ask:
What do you use these for?
How old are these?
Where did you get these from?
Are you happy with them?

Present refractive correction-contact lenses
If unsure, ask: Do you wear contact lenses?
If yes, ask:
When did you first start wearing contact lenses?
What type of lenses do you wear?
How old are these?
Where did you get these from?
For how many hours do you wear these?
How many days per week?
Do you ever wear them for longer?
What cleaning solutions do you use?
When was your last aftercare?
When is the next?
Are you happy with these lenses?
How long have you worn them today?

Present refractive correction-low vision aids
If older patient with poor vision, ask: Do you use a magnifier or any other device to help you read or watch TV?
If yes, then for each device ask:
When did you first start using this?
What do you use it for?
Can you show me how you use it?
Where did you get it from?
Are you happy using this?
If from a hospital based low vision clinic ask: When is your next hospital appointment?

Previous eye treatment
Ask: Have you ever had any eye injuries, infections, surgery or other treatment? And: Have you ever had vision training (eye exercises) or eye patching?
For each reported treatment ask:
What were you treated for?
How long ago was this?
Where did you have this treatment?
Are you still receiving this treatment?
If yes, ask: When is your next appointment?
When was your last eye examination?

General health
Ask about:
Medical history
Medication
Allergies and hypersensitivities
Last medical examination.
Explain: I need to know about your general health as it can affect your eyes.
The patient may feel that their general health is okay, despite having a borderline illness or one controlled by medicine.
So, ask: Any high blood pressure, diabetes or anything else?
For each treatment reported ask:
How long have you had this?
Who is treating you?
When was your last check-up?
When is your next check-up?

Systemic diseases, such as, diabetes, systemic hypertension, arthritis and thyroid disorders have ocular manifestations.

Medication
Explain: Medicine can also affect your eyes. Ask: Are you taking any medicine, eye drops or pills?
The patient may not consider that drops that whiten the eyes, hay fever pills or contraceptive pills are medication.
Ask: Can you tell me the name of the medicine you take and how often you take it? Do you have a written list of these?
Medicines and side effects are referenced in the British National Formulary – http://www.bnf.org.
Many systemic medications can have ocular side effects or may interact with the topical diagnostic drugs optometrists use.

Allergies and drug hypersensitivity
Ask: Do you suffer from any allergies? And: Have you ever had a bad reaction to medicine or eye drops?'

Allergies can cause eye irritation and influence tolerance to contact lenses; drug hypersensitivity may occur with topical diagnostic drugs used by optometrists.

Family ocular history
Ask: Has anybody in your family had any eye problems such as lazy eye or glaucoma?

Some eye abnormalities are inherited:

The prevalence of strabismus is
~ 1% if neither parent has strabismus
~ 10-20% if one parent has strabismus
~ 30-40% if both parents have strabismus.

The prevalence of primary open angle glaucoma (POAG) is:

~ 1% in the general population aged over 40 years
~ 10-20% if a parent or sibling has POAG.

Family medical history
Ask: Has anybody in your family had any medical problems such as high blood pressure or diabetes?

Some systemic diseases that show ocular manifestations are hereditary.

The prevalence of systemic hypertension is:

~ 3% if neither parent has systemic hypertension
~ 25% if one parent has systemic hypertension
~ 40% if both parents have systemic hypertension.

The prevalence of non-insulin dependent diabetes (NIDDM) is:

~ 2% in the general population
~ 4-10% if one parent has NIDDM
~ 5-35% if both parents have NIDDM
~ 3-11% if a sibling has NIDDM.

Occupation, hobbies and driving
Ask: What is your occupation? Do you play sports regularly? Do you have any hobbies? Do you drive?

What are patient's visual demands? Does the patient use safety eyewear (occupation, sports)? Has the patient considered using contact lenses for football, rugby? Does the patient need separate spectacles (computer screen, hobbies)? Does the patient have a pair of glasses if he/she uses contact lenses for driving?

Hints and tips
The case history continues throughout the examination.

Reviewing previous records is advised but do not assume that information from a previous case history is still current.
Conduct the case history in a logical order to avoid repeating questions.
Be in control as otherwise the case history may overrun.
Record positive and negative patient responses.
From the legal viewpoint, no recorded response means question was not asked.
Use only universally accepted abbreviations.
Remember that the patient's record is confidential.
Complete records with the expectation that they could be read by somebody else:
Another optometrist in your practice.
An optometrist from elsewhere auditing your records for clinical and/or financial reasons.
A lawyer.

In the final discussion at end of examination, review findings with regard to the chief complaint and associated symptoms.

Reassure the patient if the cause of a problem remains unknown at the end of the examination.
Explain what has been ruled out especially for a patient with a family ocular history of hereditary eye diseases.

If the patient complains of headaches, it is important to ask whether the headaches wake the patient during the night as these headaches are likely to have a serious cause.

If diplopia is a presenting symptom they it is necessary to note whether it is recent or longstanding, whether it occurs at distance or near, methods of overcoming the diplopia, mode of onset:

- Sudden may mean a palsy
- Gradual may mean decompensation.
- For a child birth history - full term, normal delivery, complications.

In the following few pages we have put together lists of questions for three categories of patients. However, history and symptoms taking will vary according with the maturation and general ability of the patient and these lists are not meant to be exhaustive or prescriptive.

History taking for a young child when the child is too young to respond directly (for example a child less than four years old)
Main reason for attending?
Any near vision or distance vision concerns from the parents?
Has a 'lazy eye' been diagnosed? If so, by whom?
If problems exist how long have they been apparent?
If these problems are longstanding, what was the age at onset?
Is there current spectacle wear?
From what age have glasses been used and what tasks were they recommended for?

Have there been any previous eye hospital visits?
Any previous ocular trauma?
Any previous patching?
Any previous or current use of prisms?
How is the general health? Any medications?
Any family history of strabismus (eye turns, in everyday language), amblyopia (lazy eye, in everyday language), refractive correction, eye operations?
At birth, was the delivery assisted?
Any birth complications?
Was the baby classed as premature?
Was the birth weight low? (≤1500 g).

Any affirmative questions with respect to the birth history should heighten the index of suspicion. For example, it is well know that children born prematurely are more likely to have eye problems.

Children who able to respond directly to questioning
Some questions will still need to be put to the parent and most answers from the child will need to be corroborated by the parent.
Main reason for attending?
Any near vision or distance vision concerns?
Any headaches? If yes, it is important to ask about their frequency, whether they occur in the morning or later in the day, whether the headaches wake the patient during the night, their duration and location.
Any eyestrain?
Any double vision? If yes, for how long, did it occur suddenly (this suggests a palsy) or gradually (this suggests decompensation) are the images side-by-side, one above the other or in between (note, some patients may not understand the terms, horizontal, vertical and oblique)? Is it with distance viewing or near viewing or both? Does it occur when looking to one side, or up or down? Any methods of overcoming it? Any idea what may have caused it?
Has a lazy eye been diagnosed? If so, by whom?
If problems exist, how long have they been apparent?
If these problems are longstanding, what was the age at onset?
Is there current spectacle wear?
From what age have glasses been used and what tasks were they recommended for?
Have there been any previous eye hospital visits?
Any previous ocular trauma?
Any previous patching?
Any previous eye exercises?
Any previous or current use of prisms?
How is the general health? Any medications?
Any family history of strabismus (eye turns, in everyday language), amblyopia (lazy eye, in everyday language), refractive correction, eye operations?
At birth, was delivery assisted?
Were there any birth complications?
Was the baby classed as premature?
Was the birth weight low? (≤1500 g)

Are there any current learning difficulties, especially with reading and writing?

History taking for adult
Any current vision or eye problems?
Main reason for attending?
Any near vision or distance vision concerns?
Are you a keen reader? If not, is this through choice or is it related to your eyes?
Any headaches? If yes, it is important to ask about the frequency, whether they occur in the morning or later in the day, whether the headaches wake the patient during the night, their duration and location.
Any eyestrain?
Any double vision? If yes, for how long, did it occur suddenly (this suggests a palsy) or gradually (this suggests decompensation) are the images side-by-side, one above the other or in between (note, some patients may not understand the terms, horizontal, vertical and oblique)? Is it with distance viewing or near viewing or both? Does it occur when looking to one side, or up or down? Any methods of overcoming it? Any idea what may have caused it?
Is there a lazy eye or an eye that doesn't see as well as the other?
If problems exist, how long have they been apparent?
If problems are longstanding, what was the age at onset?
Is there current spectacle wear?
From what age have glasses been used and what tasks were they recommended for?
Have there been any previous eye hospital visits?
Any previous ocular trauma?
Any previous patching?
Any previous eye exercises?
Any previous or current use of prisms?
How is the general health? Any medications?
Any family ocular history of strabismus (eye turns, in in everyday language), amblyopia (lazy eye, in in everyday language), refractive correction, eye operations, glaucoma, cataract, age-related macular degeneration?
Any family medical history of hypertension, diabetes (insulin dependent or none insulin dependent), heart disease, thyroid problems?

Recording findings

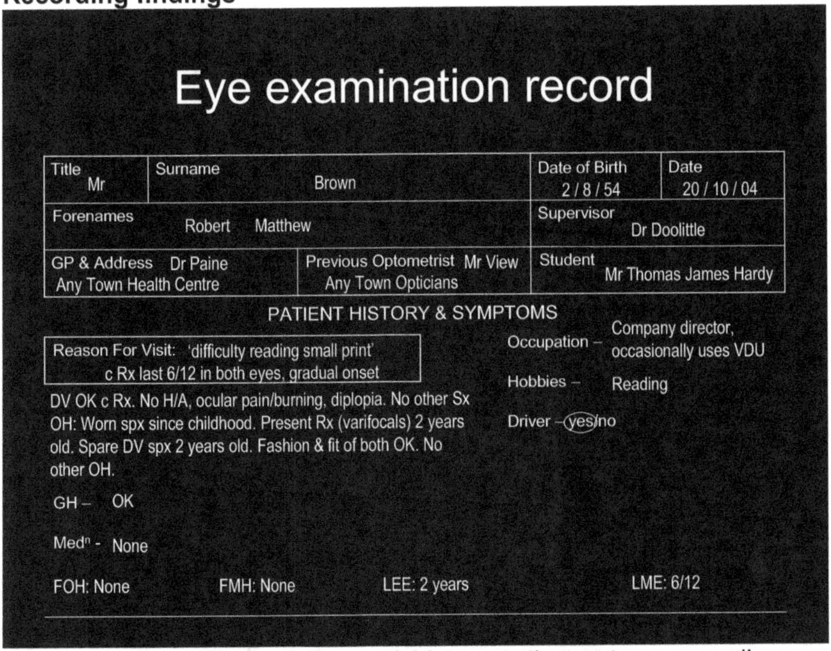

Eye examination record

Title	Surname		Date of Birth	Date
Mr	Brown		2 / 8 / 54	20 / 10 / 04
Forenames	Robert Matthew		Supervisor	Dr Doolittle
GP & Address Dr Paine Any Town Health Centre	Previous Optometrist Mr View Any Town Opticians		Student	Mr Thomas James Hardy

PATIENT HISTORY & SYMPTOMS

Reason For Visit: 'difficulty reading small print'
c Rx last 6/12 in both eyes, gradual onset

Occupation – Company director, occasionally uses VDU

Hobbies – Reading

DV OK c Rx. No H/A, ocular pain/burning, diplopia. No other Sx
OH: Worn spx since childhood. Present Rx (varifocals) 2 years old. Spare DV spx 2 years old. Fashion & fit of both OK. No other OH.

Driver – yes/no

GH – OK

Med^n - None

FOH: None   FMH: None   LEE: 2 years   LME: 6/12

Figure 1 Example history and symptoms recording

Abbreviations: c̄ –with; Rx–prescription; DV–distance vision; Sx symptoms; spx–spectacles; OH–ocular history; GH–general health; Med^n–medication; FOH–family ocular history; FMH–family medical history; LEE–last eye examination; LME–last medical examination.

Chapter 2 Measurement of visual acuity

Introduction
In the eye care field, vision is often described as the smallest symbol or letter that can be identified without the use of an optical device such as spectacles or contact lenses. Visual acuity (VA) can be described as the smallest symbol or letter that can be identified with the aid of an optical device such as spectacles or contact lenses. For reasons of simplicity and brevity we will refer only to VA in this chapter although the reader should remember that vision and VA are different entities.

Use
Accurate VA assessment is important in terms of detecting and monitoring disease, determining the outcome of refraction and for choosing targets to use in cover testing. Visual acuity can be measured with a Snellen chart or any system that uses letters or symbols (also known as optotypes) can be described as assessing recognition or identification (minimum recognisable) ability. Tests that use preferential looking such as the Keeler Acuity or Cardiff Acuity charts can be described as assessing resolution (minimum resolvable) ability. All VA charts record an estimate of the VA; this depends on several factors including the actual VA, motivation and attention of the patient, the presence of any pathology and the skill of the practitioner.

Procedure
For most patients VA should be measured with each eye in turn, testing the suspect eye first (if there is one) and then binocularly; this will depend on cooperation. If there is some suspicion that one eye sees poorly perhaps from a health visitor, school nurse or orthoptic screening referral letter then the suspect eye should be tested first.

Even young children are quite capable of remembering letters from one eye to the next so different letters of approximate equal difficulty should be used for each VA determination. Occlusion of one eye for a young child in order to carry out monocular VA assessment is probably best achieved by sitting the child on the mother's lap and asking the mother to cover each eye in turn. An alternative is to use a lightweight child's spectacle frame glazed with an occluder or frosted lens on one side. For older children it is better to use a hand held occluder such as a cover stick or an occluding trial lens placed in the trial frame. It is not appropriate to ask the patient to cover one eye with the palm of their hand as some patients may peak between their fingers or press too firmly, distort the cornea and lead to an artificially reduced VA measurement when that eye is assessed.

There are several different types of VA chart; perhaps the most commonly used are the standard 6 m Snellen chart with a mirror, the Sheridan Gardiner test and the logMAR Acuity Test (also known as Keeler Crowded/Uncrowded Cards); all can be used with or without matching cards. For many young children it is not possible to use the 6m Snellen chart with a mirror since the mirror may confuse them, or they may just turn around and look at the chart.

Single letters are easier to identify correctly than letters arranged in groups; with single letters there is less contour interaction and the crowding phenomenon is reduced. Pointing to one letter on a line of letters with a finger also reduces contour interaction and therefore makes the task easier than reading the line without pointing. Finger pointing should be noted on the record card as a memo that the child did not achieve grouped letter VA.

All patients no matter what the age should be encouraged to guess letters especially if they read a line of letters quickly and accurately and then stop. Forcing patients to their VA threshold will make the measurement more accurate (forced choice) as many patients will go onto read another line or line and a half quite well. Patients should be encouraged and allowed to guess but not allowed to lean or move forward. For older people with VA poorer than 6/60 in one or both eyes, a single 6/60 letter printed onto white paper can used to assess VA. The practitioner can position the letter at the appropriate distance and easily measure VA without asking the patient to move from the chair.

For more detailed information about the tests described below the reader is referred to the instruction booklet that accompanies each test.

Distance VA tests
Snellen

This was the first standardised VA chart and was developed in 1862. Probably the most widely used chart, it is quick and easy to use, familiar to clinicians and patients worldwide and correlates well with patient's subjective VA in most but not all cases.

However, the Snellen chart does suffer with many well-documented design problems.
Some letters are easier to see than others, especially when small.
Relative legibility of letters will depend on the magnitude and axis of any uncorrected astigmatism.
Many charts fail to adhere to the recommendations and standards relating to the selection of letters.
Most charts have one 6/60 letter and an increasing number of letters on lower lines. Patients with poor VA are required to read fewer letters than those with good VA. The small number of large letters limits the charts usefulness when assessing people with very poor VA.
Letters on lower lines are more crowded than those towards the top of the chart and crowding increases the task difficulty, therefore the visual demand changes down the chart.
Spacing between each letter and each row of letters bears no systematic relationship to the width and height or letters.

For this reason, VA measured at a distance of less than 6m cannot easily be equated to a 6m equivalent.

Most Snellen charts are designed to be used with a mirror to provide a 6m working distance; the concept of how a mirror works can be confusing for many young children.

The progression of letter sizes follows an approximate geometrical progression with letter size doubling every other line.

Progression is irregular with extra lines at the bottom and lines omitted at the top. Statistical analyses of results are precluded and therefore the chart has very little use in modern eye care research.

VA is noted as the lowest line of letters read. In practice patients seldom read all of one line and no letters on the line below and sometimes the endpoint may spread over three lines.

For example, the result 6/6-3+2 is difficult to convey and could easily be noted as 6/9+4+2.

There are no agreed standards for this type of notation and there is ample room for confusion.

Clues to active pathology can be missed.

For example, a patient that has a best-corrected VA of 6/7.5 will be measured as 6/9 since most Snellen charts do not have a 6/7.5 line.

If at the next examination the VA has reduced to 6/9 due to active pathology then this will be missed because the examiner would not realise there had been any VA change.

Recording findings
R 6/36, L 6/9, B 6/9 Snellen.

Expected findings
For a young adult, R 6/5, L 6/5, B 6/5 Snellen.
For an older adult, R 6/6, L 6/6, B 6/6 Snellen.

LogMAR
This chart was designed to overcome many of the shortcomings of the Snellen chart. There are several different versions of this chart but all adhere to original principles described by Bailey and Lovie in 1976 and all work in the same way. Internal (back lit) and external illuminated versions are available.

Five letters on each line.

Spacing between each letter and each row is related to the width and height of the letters respectively.

Each row is a scaled down version of the row above.

The task remains the same as the patient reads down the chart and therefore results obtained at different viewing distances can easily be equated.

The progression of letter sizes is uniform, increasing in a constant ratio of 1.26 (0.1 log unit steps).

The result is noted in terms of a logMAR score (log minimum angle of resolution); 6/6 is equivalent to a logMAR of zero ($\log_{10}$ of 1=0) and 6/60 is equivalent to 1 ($\log_{10}$ of 10=1).

Smaller letters have a negative logMAR score since log10 of any number less than one is negative.
Large letters have a positive score.
As letter size changes in units of 0.1 log units per row, each letter has been assigned a score of 0.02 (5 letters on each line).
The final logMAR score takes into account every letter that has been read correctly, no matter which line it was read from.
However, as with the Snellen chart contour interaction is not equal across each line and the letters at each end will be easier to identify.

Recording findings
R 0.00, L 0.12, B 0.02 logMAR.

Expected findings
For a young adult, R −0.10, L −0.10, B −0.12 logMAR.
For an older adult, R −0.10, L −0.10, B −0.12 logMAR.

Keeler Crowded/Uncrowded cards
This chart comprises three sets of cards and a key card for letter matching in patients who are unable to name letters.
Two sets are designed to measure crowded linear VA and are identical apart from differing arrangement of letters, while the third set consists of cards with two widely spaced uncrowded letters on each card.
The test is usually performed at a distance of 3 m in a well-illuminated room.
There are four letters on each line (chosen from six XVOHUY) of approximately equal legibility with all letters being symmetrical about the vertical midline.
The visual demand on each line is constant.
Each line on the chart represents a change of 0.1 log units in acuity level and each letter has a value of 0.025 log unit.
At 3m the chart and the examiner are more likely to be within the sphere of interest of the child. Measured VA ranges from 6/38 to 6/3 at 3 m.
The initial letter VA level can be determined using the screening cards (cards 1 to 3 in each of the crowded tests).
The last successful response on the screening cards is used to determine the starting point for the measurement of linear VA.
Using this technique an estimation of the patients VA can be made and then refined quickly, as it is not necessary for all the test cards to be used.
The test is very portable and low cost but needs good external illumination.
VA can be recorded in metric Snellen, logMAR and modified logMAR (reciprocal of logMAR) notation.

Recording findings
R 6/12, L 6/6, B 6/6 Keeler Crowded.

Expected findings
For a young adult, R 6/5, L 6/5, B 6/5 Keeler Crowded.
For an older adult, R 6/6, L 6/6, B 6/6 Keeler Crowded.

Sheridan-Gardiner

This test is designed to assess VA in young or mentally challenged patients.
It consists of five booklets containing single letter optotypes on each page.
Three booklets assess VA from 6/60 to 6/18, 6/18 to 6/6 and 6/6 to 6/3 respectively with three letters at each VA level to prevent familiarisation of the letters confounding the results.
The fourth booklet has one letter at each VA level and can be used to assess VA from 6/60 to 6/6.
The test is designed to be used at 6m but may be used at 3m by halving the VA values or at 6m using a mirror.
There is also a booklet for measuring reduced Snellen and near VA in N notation.

Recording findings

R 6/12, L 6/6, B 6/6 Sheridan-Gardner.

Expected findings

For a young adult, R 6/5, L 6/5, B 6/5 Sheridan-Gardner.
For an older adult, R 6/6, L 6/6, B 6/6 Sheridan-Gardner.

Kay Pictures

This chart is designed for young children who are unfamiliar with letters (2 to 5 years of age) and may also be useful when assessing mentally challenged people of any age.
The test consists of easily recognisable shapes e.g. a house, with one shape on each page; a 'recognition booklet' is provided to help determine how the child interprets each shape.
For example, the house shape may be interpreted as home or school.
This information can then be used when the test is conducted.
There are 3m and 6m versions with metric and Snellen notation as well as 3m logMAR versions with single and crowded letters.
A disadvantage of the test is that it uses single optotypes and therefore has no crowding effects.

Recording findings

R 6/12, L 6/6, B 6/6 Kay Pictures.

Expected findings

For a child, R 6/6, L 6/6, B 6/6 Kay Pictures.

LH distance acuity symbols

This chart is suitable for children aged 18 months and above and is available in both single and crowded formats.
The symbols are uniform in detail, line width and overall size providing a more standardised VA task.
The test is based on four symbols house, heart (or apple) and square, which blur equally, that is, all symbols are equally sensitive to blur and equally difficult to distinguish.
This means when blurred all the symbols appear to the observer to be circles.

The patient can still perceive answering 'correctly', while the examiner can easily detect the VA threshold without revealing to the child the failure of not recognising the symbol.
The symbols are easy to name, sign or point to on a key card or with the help of separate response cards or 3D symbols that match the chart symbols in appearance.
Versions with internal (back light) or external illumination are available.

Recording findings
R 6/9, L 6/6, B 6/6 LH symbols.

Expected findings
For a child, R 6/6, L 6/6, B 6/6 LH symbols.

Cardiff Acuity Cards
These cards are designed to measure VA in children aged 1 to 3 years but can be used in older children and adults with intellectual impairment.
The targets are described as vanishing optotypes and consist of a white band boarded by two black bands, each half the width of the white band and all on a neutral grey background.
The average illuminance of the target is equal to that of the grey background.
If the target lies beyond the subject's VA limit, it merges with the grey background and becomes invisible.
The targets are all of the same size but the black and white bands decrease in width.
VA is recorded as the narrowest white band for which the target is visible.
The test uses the principle of preferential looking; an infant will choose to look towards a target rather than towards a plain stimulus.
The cards are held with a vertical orientation in front of the child at either 50 cm or 1 m depending on where the child's attention can be obtained (a working distance of 1 m is recommended whenever possible).
It is important that the examiner is unaware of the location of the target (bottom or top) and should present each card without looking at the front where the optotypes are printed.
The examiner judges in which direction the child is looking (up or down).
For any given target width if the examiner incorrectly estimates the target position, or is unable to make a judgement form the child's responses then the target is assumed to be beyond the child's VA limit.
Three cards are included at each VA level although only two are usually presented.
Once one card has been presented neither child or examiner can predict the position of the next card to be presented.
The vertical orientation of the card allows easier discrimination in cases of nystagmus.
If the direction of gaze of the child and the position of the target are the same another card with finer lines is presented.
The endpoint is taken as the highest level at which least two out of three cards are scored correctly.
At 1 m the VA range measured is 6/60 to 6/6 and at 50 cm the range is 6/120 to 6/12.

Recording findings
R 6/18, L 6/12, B 6/12 Cardiff cards.

Expected findings
For a child, R 6/6, L 6/6, B 6/6 Cardiff cards.

Keeler Acuity Cards
This is a grating preferential looking test.
The patterns utilized are square wave gratings described in terms of their spatial frequency i.e. the number of black and white pairs in each degree of visual angle. The higher the spatial frequency the finer the grating.
The grating is placed in a circle with a white border; in order to prevent edge effects confounding the results there is also an empty circle on the grey side of the card.
The stimulus must be isoluminant (equal average luminance) to the blank stimulus. When the stimulus is beyond the resolution of limit of the viewer the card will appear to have two grey patches of equal luminance within the white circles under these circumstances the infant will show no looking preference.
This design feature ensures that the VA estimate is based on the ability to detect and resolve the grating rather than a preference for one shade of grey over another.
Gratings of increased spatial frequency are presented to an infant and their looking responses recorded.
The highest spatial frequency (finest grating) that elicits an appropriate looking response is used to estimate VA.

Grating and preferential looking tests tend to give a higher acuity than a letter test simply because the observer is required only to resolve the target and not to identify it.

Recording findings
R 6/18, L 6/12, B 6/12 Keeler acuity cards.

Expected findings
For a child, R 6/6, L 6/6, B 6/6 Keeler acuity cards.

Near reading acuity and visual acuity
Faculty of Ophthalmologists chart
This is a chart used in many optometric practices.
As it consists of words in context and not individual letters it does not assess near VA but near reading acuity.
It uses N notation; the number following the N corresponds to point size, with one point being equal to 1/72 of an inch.
The range is from N5 to N48 and there are various versions with various passages of text.
Patients are not tested to threshold as N5 is approximately equivalent to 6/9 at 25 cm.
Pathology can be missed, for example if a patient has N3 reading acuity at 35 cm this will be recorded as N5 at 35 cm.

If the patient later presents with subtle retinal disease and the reading acuity at 35 cm has decreased to N5, the practitioner will be unaware of this clinically significant change.

The chart has also been criticized for not simulating a real world task, because of the high contrast between the letters and the background.

Reading acuity should be recorded monocularly and binocularly and any asymmetry noted.

Most versions also have music, classified ads and technical drawings therefore some functional testing is possible.

It is common practice to assess the near reading acuity with the use of additional localised lighting. A reduction in reading speed when the lamp is switched off can be used to demonstrate the importance of localised lighting to older people.

A requirement of many patients is to be able to read newspaper-sized print; N8 is approximately equivalent to column newspaper print in size but probably not contrast.

It is important to ask the individual to read out loud since an inter-ocular change in reading speed or accuracy may indicate macular dysfunction.

The preferred reading distance should be measured to the nearest 1 cm and recorded with the N number that corresponds to the smallest size of print read. An N number without reading distance is a measurement of size and not reading acuity. This applies to all reading acuity and near VA charts.

Recording findings
R N6 at 25 cm, L N5 at 25 cm, B N5 at 30 cm, Faculty Ophthal.

Expected findings
R N5 at 40 cm, L N5 at 40 cm, B N5 at 40 cm, Faculty Ophthal.

Maclure reading chart and bar reading book
This can be used to measure reading acuity in young children.
The reading material has been chosen by a specialist in the teaching of reading and is based on the reading ability to be expected for different age groups of children. Each age has been given a grade, numbered 1 to 7, so that even if a child's reading ability is not equal to the average age, the grade number can be used to give an indication of the reading acuity.
Within each grade, specimens of printing in sizes N5 to N48 have been used.
The chart attempts to relate text to age. The text structure changes in terms of word and line length and difficulty.
Each book also contains a 6 m distance chart with lower case or 'school script letters', a standard 6 m Snellen chart and reduced Snellen and 'school script' distance charts that must be used at 35 cm.

Recording findings
R N6 at 20 cm, L N6 at 20 cm, B N5 at 20 cm, Maclure.

Expected findings
R N5 at 25 cm, L N5 at 25 cm, B N5 at 25 cm, Maclure.

LogMAR near visual acuity letter chart
This is very similar in design to the logMAR distance acuity test with 5 letters on each of 17 lines.
The chart has all the advantages associated with a logMAR design (see above) and also the one disadvantage, less crowding at the end of each line of letters.
As the chart is comprised of individual letters it does measure near visual acuity and not reading acuity.
Near VA can be recorded in terms M units (1M corresponding to the resolution of a 5 degree target at 1m and roughly corresponds to newspaper sized print), decimal, reduced Snellen (metric and imperial).
In order for the VA values printed on the card to be valid the working distance has to be 40 cm.
The chart is usually printed on both sides with a different series of letters to avoid the learning effects when right and left and binocular VA is measured.

Recording findings
R 0.10, L 0.12, B 0.10 at 40 cm, near logMAR.

Expected findings
R – 0.10, L – 0.10, B – 0.14 at 40 cm, near logMAR.

LH symbols near acuity chart
This is very similar in design to the LH distance acuity chart and uses the same house, heart (or apple), circle and square symbols.
For young children it is probably better to attempt a binocular near visual acuity (to build confidence) measurement before going on to monocular near VA.

Recording findings
R 0.10, L 0.12, B 0.10 at 40 cm, LH near symbols.

Expected findings
R – 0.10, L – 0.10, B – 0.14 at 40 cm, LH near symbols.

Institute of Optometry (IOO) near test card
This chart builds on recent research on visual acuity assessment yet retains a fairly familiar appearance.
It is easy to use for clinicians who are accustomed to conventional designs.
Produced as an A5 size laminated card.
It consists of a column of isolated words and allows a rapid estimate of visual acuity.
The words are simple and can be read by young or poor readers and are arranged in random order with a logarithmic progression in size.
The chart uses point size units, e.g. N6.
A conversion table is included enabling point size to be converted to logMAR, decimal, imperial Snellen and metric Snellen notation.

Recording findings
R N6 at 20 cm, L N6 at 20 cm, B N5 at 20 cm, IOO.

Expected findings
R N5 at 25 cm, L N5 at 25 cm, B N5 at 25 cm, IOO.

Practical near acuity chart (PNAC)
This is a single card with a print size range from N80 to N5, with a regular decreasing progression of 0.1 logMAR, with high contrast lower-case Times Roman font, and N, M (1M is equivalent to N8) and logMAR notation.
The logMAR values printed on the card are valid only when the testing distance is 25 cm.
There are 13 rows with three related words per row.
Each row has one three-letter, one four letter and one five letter word, totalling 12 letters.
When using the logMAR notation, each three- and four-letter word should be scored at 0.03 log units, and each five-letter word at 0.40 log units (adding 0.10 log units for each line).
When using N notation, the patient can be asked to hold the card at their habitual reading distance; this then needs to be noted along with the N value for the smallest words read.
The word reading threshold is reached when fewer than two words on a row are read correctly.
Several word sequences for the chart are available to reduce learning effects with repetition.
The words have been chosen to be easily recognisable by people with the educational ability of an average 9 year old.
The reverse side of the card contains commonly used print sizes, so fluency and reading speed can be tested once near visual acuity threshold has been established.

Recording findings
R N6 at 35 cm, L N6 at 30 cm, B N5 at 35 cm, PNAC.

Expected findings
R N5 at 33 cm, L N5 at 33 cm, B N5 at 33 cm, PNAC.

Hints and tips
Use the most complex chart that the patient can cope with.
Determine the VA threshold by forcing the patient to guess when they are uncertain of letters.
Record VA monocularly and binocularly, include the working distance for near measurements and note the type of test used.

Pinhole test
Introduction
This is a trial case accessory and consists of an occluder with a hole in the middle usually 1 to 2 mm in diameter.

Use
The pinhole test is used to determine whether reduced VA is due to refractive error or ocular disease. The pinhole reduces effect of ametropic blur by reducing effective pupil size. If the VA improves with the pinhole test then the reduced VA is due to uncorrected refractive error; if the VA does not improve with the pinhole test then the reduced VA is due to ocular disease.

Procedure
Place pinhole occluder in front of eye with reduced vision.
Ask patient to move eye and head until some letters can be read on the letter chart.
Ask patient to read the lowest line of letters they can see looking through the pinhole.

Recording findings
RV6/12, NIPH - patient has unaided vision of 6/12 in the R eye that is not improved with a pinhole i.e. reduction is due to ocular disease and will not improve even with the optimum refractive correction.

RV6/12, 6/6 PH – patient has unaided vision of 6/12 in the R eye that improves to 6/6 with a pinhole i.e. reduction is due to uncorrected refractive error and will improve with optimum refractive correction.

Chapter 3 Focimetry of a cylindrical lens

Introduction
It is often useful to determine the power of unknown lenses. This can be done using hand neutralisation, or with a focimeter.

Use
Focimetry can be used to determine the back vertex power of a lens, any prismatic effect, and also the orientation of the lens within a spectacle frame. Focimeters will generally have one of two types of target, either a ring of dots (corona, or European) or a crossed lines target (American).

The ring of dots target consists of a small ring of dots over a graticule with standard axis notation reading from 0° to 180° anticlockwise. When a spherical lens is being measured, the ring of dots will be blurred when out of focus, and crisp when in focus, at which time the power of the lens can be read off the power wheel. When an astigmatic lens is being measured, the dots will be drawn out into two focal lines (at different powers). The power should be recorded twice (once for the sphere and once for the cyl), at the positions at which the dots are drawn into the sharpest lines. For each power, there will be a corresponding axis, which can be read off the graticule.

The crossed line target consists of two sets of lines crossed at 90° to each other. In some models, each set of lines must be rotated and aligned with one of the principal meridians of the lens before a sharp image can be obtained.

Procedure
Focusing the eyepiece
Place a piece of paper between the lens stop and the telescope objective.
Observe whether or not the graticule lines are in focus. If they are then no further adjustments need to be made.
If they are not in focus, turn the eyepiece anticlockwise until the lines are blurred. Then turn the eyepiece clockwise until the lines are sharply focussed.
Switch the instrument on and place the power wheel at zero.
The focimeter target should be clear.
If the target is not clear, then the instrument may need to be recalibrated.
Measuring a spherical lens
Place the back surface of the lens against the lens rest.
Release the lens holder so that it secures the lens against the lens stop.
Position the lens so that the target is as near to the centre of the graticule as possible.
Rotate the lens wheel until the target becomes clear.

Note the power from the drum.

Measuring an astigmatic lens with a crossed line focimeter
Position the lens so that the target is as near to the centre of the graticule as possible.
Turn the power wheel until one of the sets of lines is sharply focussed as possible.
If the instrument requires it, rotate the target to see whether the sharpness increases when the target is aligned with the appropriate meridian.
Otherwise, turn the dial just below the eyepiece to move the graticule in line with the focussed lines and read the axis of the protractor scale.
Repeat for the other set of lines.

Measuring an astigmatic lens with a ring of dots focimeter
Position the lens so that the target is as near as possible to the centre of the graticule.
Turn the power wheel until the ring of dots stretches out to form a set of lines in one direction.
Make a note of the power from the power wheel.
Turn the dial just below the eyepiece until the graticule is in line with the focussed 'lines' and read the axis off the protractor scale.
Repeat, but focus the dots so that they form sharp lines at 90° to the axis recorded.

Hints and tips
The prescription written down will now be in the following form (the following are examples):

+ 4.00 along 70 degree meridian.
+ 8.00 along the 160 degree meridian.
You can choose to write this in plus or minus cyl form.
+ 4.00 / + 4.00 x 160, or
+ 8.00 / - 4.00 x 70.

A quicker way may be to follow these steps:

- ➢ Take the first power reading as the sphere
- ➢ No need to record the axis
- ➢ Take the second power reading to be the cyl
- ➢ Record the axis of the second meridian
- ➢ Check the approximate powers before writing anything down.
- ➢ If working in minus cyl ensure that the first meridian recorded (the sphere) is the most positive one.

Chapter 4 Brückner test

Introduction
This test is used to assess the symmetry of binocular fixation by comparing the brightness of the red reflex in each of the two eyes using a direct ophthalmoscope. It can be used as a pre-refraction test or as a specialist binocular vision test.

Use
This test is mainly used in infants, young children and patients with limited co-operation and can be used to screen for strabismus, anisometropia, media opacities, and posterior pole abnormalities.

Procedure
The purpose of this test is to assess the symmetry of binocular fixation by comparing the brightness of the red reflex in each of the two eyes and is particularly useful for very young patients with limited co-operation.

Instruct the patient to remove any refractive correction.
Dim room lights.
Direct the ophthalmoscope toward the patient's eyes from a distance of 80 to 100 cm using a large round patch of light to illuminate both pupils simultaneously.
Instruct the patient to look at the centre of the light.
Look through the peephole of the ophthalmoscope and dial in the lens that gives a clear view of the patient's pupils.
While observing the Hirschberg reflexes against the red reflex in the pupil, the brightness of each red reflex can be compared.
If the two reflexes are equally bright, there is binocular fixation.
If the reflexes are not equally bright, the darker red reflex indicates the fixing eye, and the brighter, lighter, or whiter reflex indicates the non-fixing eye.
The difference in brightness may be caused by strabismus, anisometropia, anisocoria, media opacities, or posterior pole abnormalities.
Note how this contrasts with the use of a retinoscope, when the reflex of an affected eye is often the darker.

Recording findings
Brückner test-R reflex brighter. See Figure 2.

Expected findings
Brückner test- equally bright reflexes R and L. See Figure 3.

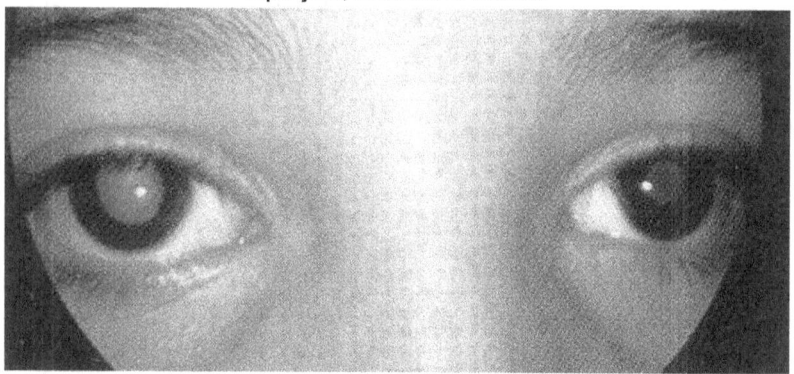

Figure 2 Brückner test-R reflex brighter.

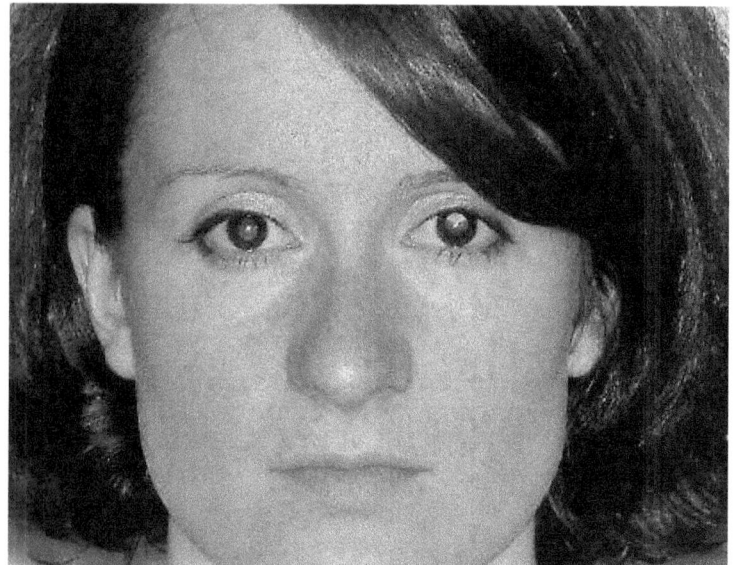

Figure 3 Brückner test- equally bright reflexes R and L.

Chapter 5 Hirschberg corneal reflexes

Introduction
This is an objective test that can be useful for assessing eye alignment in paediatric cases.

Use
Useful in paediatric cases when the patient is not co-operative enough for a cover test and the practitioner needs to differentiate between a pseudo-strabismus and a strabismus.

Procedure
Room lights on.
Hold penlight in front of 40-50cm from the patient.
Shine light on to the eyes so both are illuminated simultaneously.
Observe position of corneal reflexes as patient views binocularly.
Reflex usually about 0.5 mm nasal to pupil centre.
Observe position of corneal reflexes in as patient views monocularly.
Fixating eye has same monocular and binocular reflex positions.
Deviating eye has different monocular and binocular reflex positions.

Recording findings
Corneal reflex shifts in the opposite direction to deviation.
Nasal shift = exotropia, temporal shift = esotropia, superior shift = hypotropia, inferior shift = hypertropia.
1 mm of decentration ≈ 22 prism dioptres (Δ) deviation.

Chapter 6 Assessment of pupil function

Introduction
Some patients with neurological problems seek the opinion of an optometrist because their condition produces symptoms that they associate with their eyes. Such symptoms include double vision, blurry vision, reduced peripheral vision, headaches and dizziness. Consequently optometrists need to be able to detect neurological disease and determine if the patient's condition warrants monitoring or treatment.

Pupil function, cranial nerve assessment and corneal sensitivity are important factors to consider in assessment for neurological disease.

Use
Assessment of pupil function can provide diagnostic information about the afferent and efferent neurological pathways responsible for pupillary and eyelid function.

Set-up
Use ambient illumination that is as dim as possible, but permits a clear view of both the patient's pupils.
Position yourself within 25 cm of the patient, but not in front of the direct line of sight.
Instruct the patient to remove spectacles if they use them.

Procedure for direct and consensual reflexes
Instruct the patient to look at the distance spotlight.
Shine the pen torch into the right eye and observe the size and speed of the pupillary constriction in this eye (the direct reflex).
Repeat step 2 two times.
Shine the light into the right eye and observe the size and the speed of the pupillary constriction in the left eye (consensual reflex).
Repeat step 4 two times.
Repeat step 2 through 5 shining the light into the left eye, again observing the direct and consensual responses of the appropriate pupils.

Procedure for swinging flash light test (relative afferent pupil defect)
With the pen torch approximately 5 cm from the eye, move the light between the eyes rapidly, leaving it on each eye for 3 to 5 seconds.
Observe the response (dilation or constriction) and the size of each pupil at the moment when the light first arrives there and during the 3 to 5 second observation period. Be sure to shine an equal intensity of light into each eye.
The swinging flashlight test should be repeated for 2 to 3 complete cycles.
Throughout the test, judge the roundness of each pupil.

If the pupils are unequal in size, perform the dim-bright pupillary test (see below for details on this).
If one or both pupils fail to respond directly or consensually, or if their responses are sluggish, test the accommodative responses of the pupil (see below).

Procedure for near or accommodative response
To test the responsiveness of the pupil to near viewing.
Tell the patient to maintain distance fixation while a target containing fine visual detail (such as a near fixation stick) is held at 10 to 40 cm from the patient Instruct the patient to look at the near target. Look for pupillary constriction.
This is known as the near or accommodative response.
Instruct the patient to return his gaze to the distance target. Look for dilation of the pupil to confirm that it had constricted during near viewing.
Repeat steps 1 to 3 if necessary to confirm the observations.

Recording findings
If all the pupillary responses are normal, write PERRLA and no MG or no RAPD (Pupils Equal Round Responsive to Light Accommodation: no Marcus Gunn or no Relative Afferent Pupillary Defect) response.
Separately describe abnormalities, such as inequality of size (anisocoria), shape, or rate of response (see also recording under dim-bright pupillary test).
If pupillary escape is observed on the swinging flashlight test, record a positive Marcus Gunn or +RAPD (positive relative afferent pupillary defect), followed by the affected eye.
Pupillary escape is observed if during the swinging flash light test as the eye is moved from one eye to the other, the pupil where the light arrives continues to dilate and not constrict as one would expect.

For example:

PERRLA, +MG L.
PRRLA, no MG, R>L by 1 mm in dim and bright light.
R: RRLA D no RAPD.
L: irregular, sluggish D and C.
R unresponsive to light direct or consensual; both pupils constrict to near; L responds to light, D and C.

Expected findings
PERRLA, no RAPD.

Note, The terms RAPD and MG are synonymous, D = direct reflex and C = consensual reflex.

Dim-bright pupillary test
Use
This test is indicated when the pupils appear to be unequal in size.

Set-up
The practitioner should be positioned directly in front of the patient slightly below the line of sight.
Ambient illumination should be low so that the only available light is that reflected from the ophthalmoscope beam.
Turn on the ophthalmoscope to full intensity and set it to the largest available beam.
Procedure
Instruct the patient to look at a distant target and not at the ophthalmoscopy light.
1. From a distance of about one metre, shine the ophthalmoscope beam onto the patient's face so that both pupils are illuminated at the same time.
2. Look through the aperture of the ophthalmoscope at the patient's pupils.
3. Orange red reflexes, due to the reflection of light from the retina, should be seen within each pupil.
4. Observing these red pupillary reflexes will enhance the ability to detect small differences in pupil size between the eyes.
5. Observe the size of each pupil, noting which eye has the larger pupil and estimating the amount of the difference in millimetres - this is the bright condition.
6. Gradually reduce the illumination level of the ophthalmoscope while observing the red reflexes and comparing the sizes of the pupils.
7. Continue to reduce the illumination until the red reflexes are barely visible.
8. Observe the size of each pupil, estimating the amount of the difference in millimetres - this is the 'dim' condition.

Repeat steps 2 through 7 one or two times to confirm the observations.

If no difference in anisocoria is observed, end the test.
If a difference in anisocoria is detected, the amount of anisocoria is quantified as follows:

Increase the room illumination until you are just able to see the pupils with unaided eyes.
Using the PD rule, measure the size of each pupil.
The size difference is the amount of anisocoria in dim illumination.
Increase the room illumination to its maximum amount.
Using the PD rule, measure the size of each pupil.
The size difference is the amount of anisocoria in bight illumination.
With the patient looking straight ahead at the fixation target, use the PD ruler to measure the size of the palpebral aperture in millimetres.
Note the position of the upper and lower lid of each eye relative to the limbus and the cornea.
Instruct the patient to fixate on your finger and have him follow it gradually into upward gaze.
Compare the intersections of the lower lids with each limbus.
Note which lid clears the limbus first or if they clear the limbus simultaneously.

Recording findings
Record the size of each pupil under bright conditions.

Record the difference in pupillary sizes (amount of anisocoria) under bright conditions.
Record the size of each pupil under dim conditions.
Record the difference in pupil size under dim conditions.
If the difference in pupil size is the same under dim and bright conditions, record 'anisocoria equal in dim and bright'. This would suggest physiological anisocoria. Record the size of the difference in millimetres. If the anisocoria changes according to the ambient lighting conditions then it is likely to be pathological.
Record the size of each palpebral aperture in millimetres in straight-ahead gaze. If the apertures were equal, and both intersect the limbus in the normal position approximately 2 millimetres below its top, record 'no ptosis of the upper lid'.
If the lower lids cleared the limbus at the same time when the patient looked upward, record 'no ptosis of lower lid'.
If one lid cleared the limbus sooner than the other, it indicates a ptosis of the more elevated lower lid.
Record 'ptosis of the lower lid' and indicate the eye whose lid cleared second.

For example:

Pupils: R>L by 0.5 mm in dim and bright, no ptosis of upper or lower lid.
Palpebral aperture: 9 mm R & L.
Pupils: in bright R = 3.5 mm, L = 3.0 mm/in dim R = 7.0 mm, L = 4.5 mm/+ ptosis upper and lower lids L.

Expected findings

Anisocoria of equal amounts under dim and bright conditions and in the absence of ptosis characterises physiological (also known as simple or essential anisocoria). It can frequently be observed in old photographs of the patient (the FAI or 'family album imaging' test).
Anisocoria more pronounced under dim conditions with a mild ptosis of the upper and lower lid in the eye with the smaller pupil, is characteristic of oculosympathetic paresis (Horner's syndrome).
Anisocoria more pronounced under bright light conditions is characteristic of dysfunction in the parasympathetic control of the pupil. If there is a ptosis in the eye with the larger pupil, a lesion of the oculomotor nerve in the eye with the larger pupil, a lesion of the oculomotor nerve (cranial nerve III) should be suspected.

Chapter 7 Cover test at distance

Introduction
The cover test is an objective dissociation test that relies on the observation of the behaviour of the eyes whilst fixation is maintained and each eye is covered and uncovered in turn. There are two main forms: cover-uncover and alternating cover.

Use
The cover test is used to elicit the presence of a heterotropia, heterophoria, orthotropia or orthophoria. It allows the direction of the deviation (horizontal, vertical, torsional or a combination) to be determined and also whether it is unilateral or alternating, constant or intermittent and the effect of refractive correction, accommodation and compensatory head posture (CHP).

Procedure
Cover-uncover test at distance

1. Patient should wear glasses if appropriate (see hints and tips below)
2. Choose the fixation target.
    a. This depends on the level of VA of each eye and the ability of the patient to follow instructions.
    b. If VA in each eye is better than 6/18 use a letter target that is one line up from the line that gives the VA in the poorer eye.
    c. If VA is <6/18 in one or both eyes a spot light is considered appropriate, although some clinicians use letter targets even with poor levels of VA but point to a specific part of the letter to aid steady fixation.
    d. A target further away than 6 m may be used when the deviation is greater at 6 m than at 33 cm.
3. Instruct the patient to: Look at this letter on the chart. Keep your eyes on the letter as I place this cover in front of your eye. If the letter appears to move, please follow it with your eyes.
4. Test patient as close as possible to the primary position of gaze to ensure that all the extra-ocular muscles are equally in tone.
5. One eye is covered and the uncovered eye is assessed for any movement to take up fixation.
6. Cover LE, observe response of RE for 2-3 seconds, if a movement is seen then the RE has a heterotropia i.e. the RE has taken up fixation while the LE is covered.
    a. Outward fixation movement means RE esotropia
    b. Inward fixation movement means RE exotropia
    c. Downward fixation movement means a hypertropia

d. Upward fixation movement means a hypotropia.
7. Uncover the LE, observe any movement of the eye behind the occluder as it is removed, and observe response of the RE for 2-3 seconds, if applicable check that the RE moves back to deviated position and note rate of recovery.
8. Cover the RE, observe response of the LE for 2-3 seconds and then as in step 4.
9. Uncover the RE and then as in step 5.
10. Estimate the size of the deviation.
    a. When a patient saccades from one end of a standard 6/9 line of letters at 6 m (on a Snellen chart to the other side, the eyes move through an angle of 2 Δ.
    b. This small movement can be used to estimate the size of deviation for a patient with a heterotropia or heterophoria i.e. how does the deviation movement compare to the saccadic movement?
    c. For example, if the deviation is five times the saccade then the deviation can be <u>estimated</u> to be 10 Δ.

See Figure 4 for cover test eye movements in a right esotropia and Figure 5 for cover test eye movements in alternating esotropia with left eye preference. Some clinicians will also check for a heterophoria when conducting the cover-uncover test.

See Figures 6 and 7 for examples of heterophoria detection using the cover-uncover test. Only do this if there is no heterotropia.

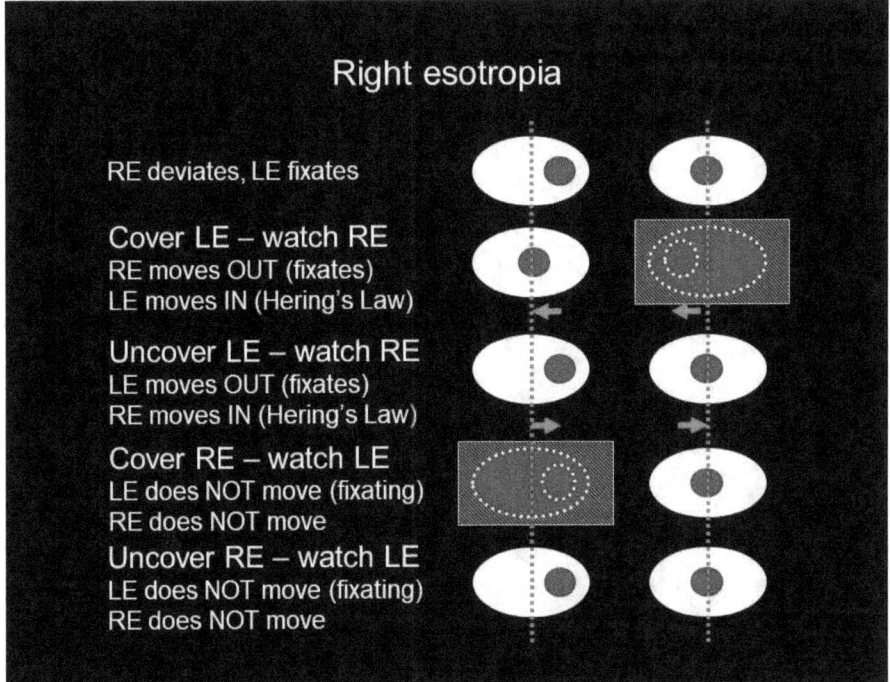

Figure 4 Cover test eye movements in right esotropia.

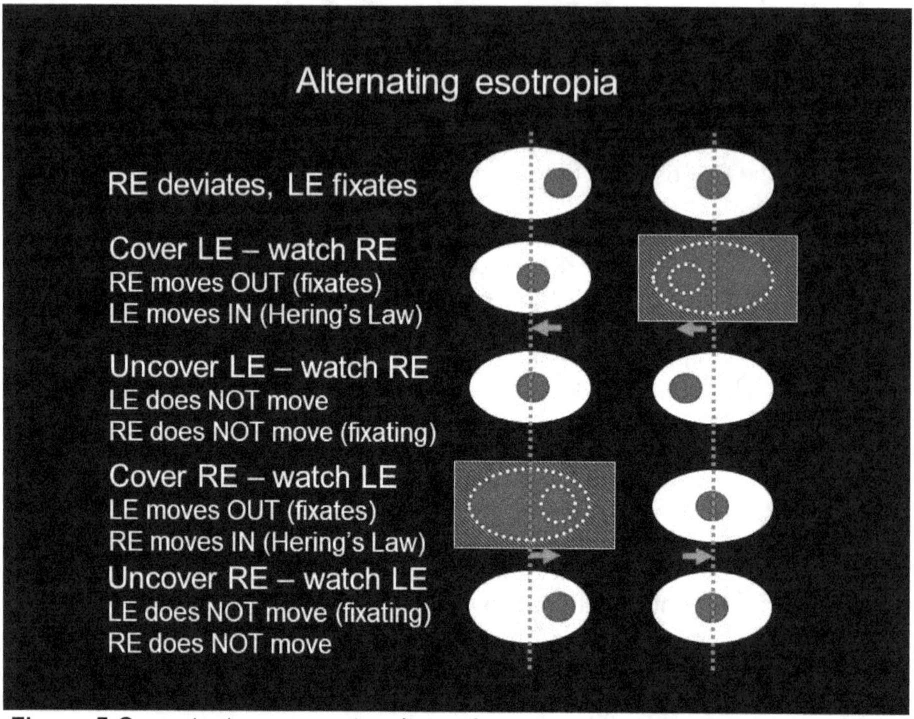

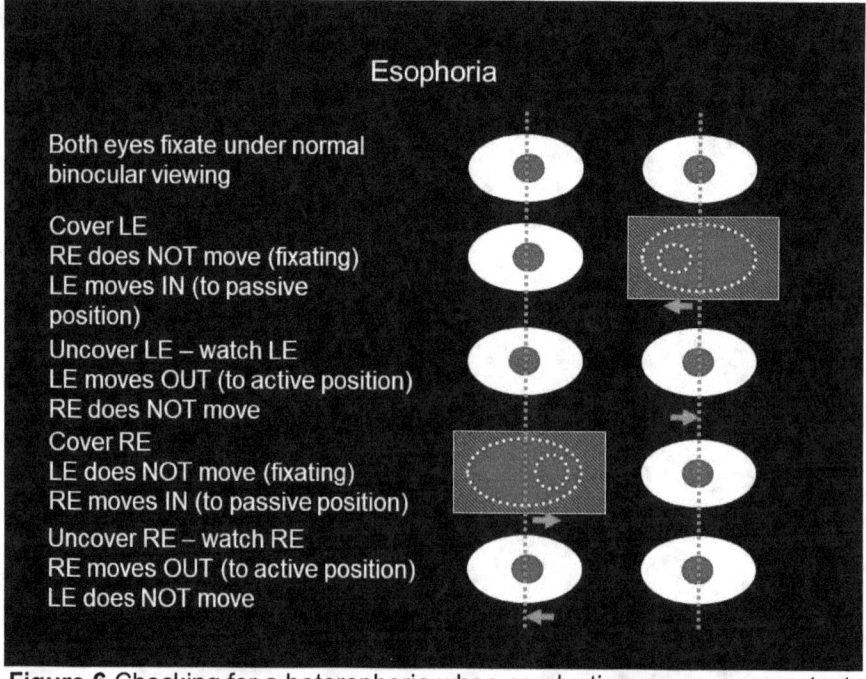

Figure 5 Cover test movements: alternating esotropia with left eye preference.

Figure 6 Checking for a heterophoria when conducting cover-uncover test.

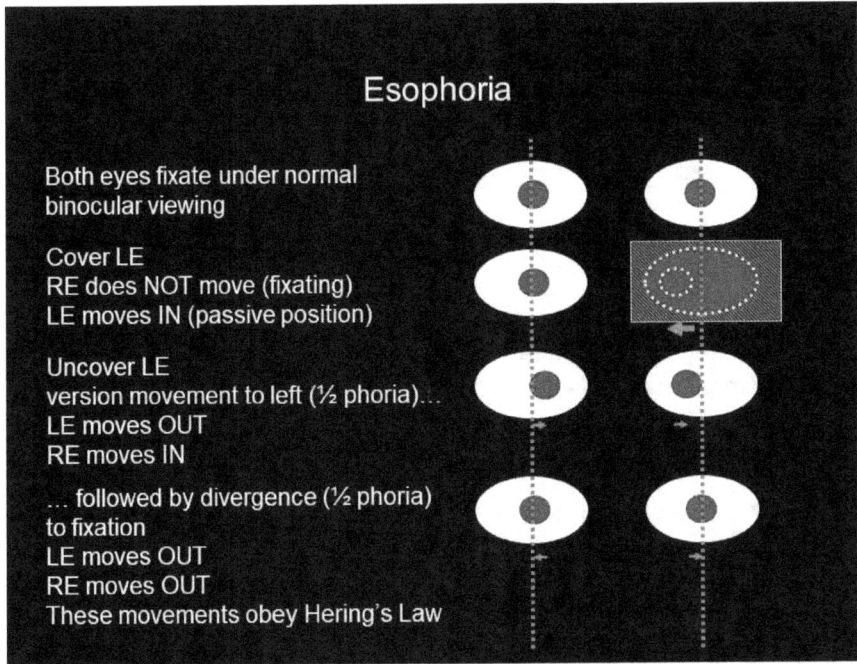

Figure 7 Checking for a heterophoria when conducting cover-uncover test.

Hints and tips
For children perform the cover test with and without any refractive correction in place.
For pre-presbyopic adults perform the cover test with and without any refractive correction in place (for myopes always use the refractive correction for a 6 m testing distance).
For presbyopic adults who require refractive correction perform the cover test with the refractive correction in place.
For all patients, if prisms are incorporated into the refractive correction then perform the cover test with and without refractive correction in place.
Perform the cover test with and without any compensatory head posture (CHP) to assess its effect on the control of the deviation.
In comprehending verbal patients ask how many targets are seen. A single image in the presence of an obvious heterotropia implies suppression.
The speed of uncovered eye to take up fixation indicates the level of vision in deviating eye e.g. slow uptake implies poor vision.
Alternating deviations indicate equal vision in each eye.
Objection to occlusion of one eye can indicate poor vision in the uncovered eye.
Manifest and latent nystagmus. Manifest nystagmus will be apparent before the occluder is introduced whereas latent nystagmus will be elicited when one eye is occluded.
Dissociated vertical divergence.
The eye behind the occluder will elevate and extort; this is very likely to be associated with latent nystagmus.
Heterophorias are normally similar in size in each eye.

Smooth and fast recovery (refixation) movements indicate that a heterophoria is compensated.
Hirschberg's reflection test.
Each mm of displacement from the centre of the cornea equates to 15Δ of deviation. This is a very gross test and should only be used if lack of patient co-operation prevents a cover test from being performed.

Alternating cover test at distance
Introduction
One eye is covered throughout the test, that is, complete dissociation is achieved and the patient is never binocular during the testing. The alternating cover test is fully dissociative and reveals the total deviation, that is, the habitual heterotropia or heterophoria experienced day-to-day by the patient. The alternating cover test follows the cover-uncover test.

Use
To elicit the presence or absence of a heterophoria along with type of deviation (eso-, exo-, hyper- and cyclophoria), effect of refractive correction, accommodation and CHP. The alternating cover test cannot differentiate between heterophoria and heterotropia but can be used to detect an intermittent heterotropia i.e. a heterophoria that changes (breaks down) to heterotropia on repeated cover testing. If the heterophoria breaks down it is likely to recover quickly during remainder of eye examination.

Procedure
1. Test the patient as close as possible to primary position of gaze to ensure that all the extra-ocular muscles are equally in tone.
2. Cover the LE for 2-3 seconds.
3. Rapidly transfer cover to the RE for 2-3 seconds, watch the LE re-fixate and make sure that that the patient never sees the target with both eyes together.
4. Rapidly transfer cover to the LE for 2-3 seconds, watch the RE re-fixate and make sure that that the patient never sees the target with both eyes together.
5. Repeat the cycle for 10-30 seconds to ensure maximum dissociation.
6. Note the rate of recovery of the covered eye when the occluder is removed.

Hints and tips
For children perform the cover test with and without any refractive correction in place.
For pre-presbyopic adults perform the cover test with and without any refractive correction in place.
For presbyopic adults who require refractive correction perform the cover test with the refractive correction in place.
For all patients, if prisms are incorporated into the refractive correction then perform the cover test with and without refractive correction in place.
Perform the cover test with and without any CHP to assess its effect on the control of the deviation.

Speed of uncovered eye to take up fixation indicates level of vision in deviating eye e.g. slow uptake implies poor vision.
Objection to occlusion of one eye can indicate poor vision in the uncovered eye.
Heterophorias are normally similar in size in both eyes.
Smooth and fast recovery (refixation) movements indicate that a heterophoria is compensated.

Other uses of the alternating cover test
In conjunction with oculo-motility testing in order to whether a deviation is comitant or incomitant and to illicit under acting and/or over acting muscle(s).
Binocular visual acuity a test used to elicit the maximum VA achieved while maintaining binocular single vision. Intermittently, a very quick cover-uncover test is performed, while the patient reads down the vision chart to determine if decompensation occurs.

Recording findings
NMD – no movement detected, 'phi' movement not assessed.
Ortho – no movement detected and no 'phi' movement.
2 SOP – no movement detected but 'phi' movement seen.
~ 4 XOP – movement estimated as 4Δ.
~ 8 SOP, slow rec. – movement estimated as 8Δ, uncompensated?
25 alt XOT with 4 RhyperT – alternating heterotropia (prism bar used).
Also record the correction worn at time of test (habitual, optimal).

Expected findings
This depends on the size of any heterotropia or heterophoria present.

Chapter 8 Cover test at near

Introduction
The cover test at near is an objective dissociation test that relies on the observation of the behaviour of the eyes whilst fixation is maintained and each eye is covered and uncovered in turn.

Use
The cover test at near is used to elicit the presence of a heterotropia, heterophoria, orthotropia or orthophoria for near fixation targets.

Procedure
As for cover-uncover test at distance steps 1-9.

10 Use a spot light target to:
  a. Observe corneal reflections. A large angle kappa may displace the corneal reflexes nasally but this displacement is symmetrical, that is, the same displacement in each eye.
  b. Highlight central, eccentric or wandering fixation.
  c. Reveal presence/absence of accommodative component to a deviation when compared to results using an accommodative stimulus.

11. Use an accommodative target to:
  a. Ensure accommodation is being exerted by using a small detailed target.
  b. Make sure each eye in turn can see the target.
  c. Reveal presence/absence of accommodative component to a deviation when compared to results using a spot light target.

Steps 10 and 11 are only useful for patients that have some accommodative amplitude.

Hints and tips
As for cover-uncover test at distance.

Chapter 9 Prism cover test

Introduction
This is an objective dissociative method of measuring the total angle of deviation using horizontal and/or vertical prisms. Torsional deviations cannot be measured using this technique.

Angles of deviation should be measured at 6 m and 33 cm in the primary position of gaze.
The test may also be used to measure deviations at different distances or fields of gaze, depending upon findings from the history, cover test and oculomotility assessment.
Results from the cover test and oculomotility assessment will provide information on the approximate size and components of the deviation, the preferred eye for fixation and whether the deviation is concomitant or incomitant.

Equipment required
Horizontal and vertical prism bars and loose square prisms.
Detailed fixation targets, selected appropriately for the age of the patient and level of visual acuity of each eye.
Occluder (for younger patients, the palm of the examiner's hand may be more suitable).

Procedure
The patient is required to fixate a target at 6 m. A prism strength approximating the size of the deviation should then be placed in front of the deviating eye in heterotropia, with the apex in the direction of the deviation, or either eye in heterophoria.
An alternate cover test should be performed, gradually increasing the prism strength until the movement of the eye is reversed. The size of the deviation is recorded as the prism value just before reversal.
The procedure should be routinely repeated for 33 cm, and, when indicated, in other fields of gaze (maintain the fixation target in the primary position while the patient's head is moved to place the eyes in the required position), fixation distances, and when fixing with each eye in the case of incomitancy.

It is essential to:

Prevent fusion and elicit the total deviation-for maximum dissociation allow sufficient time (at least two seconds) for the patient to fixate the target accurately, followed by a quick movement of the occluder to the other eye.

Maintain and control accommodation by using a detailed fixation target appropriate for the patient's age.

Simultaneous prism cover test
Introduction
This is a modification of the prism cover test and is used to measure the heterotropic component of a deviation that has heterotropic and heterophoric components, for instance in some cases of microtropia. Assessment of the size of the heterotropia enables more accurate classification of the type of deviation.

Procedure
The prism is placed in front of the deviating eye and a cover-uncover test is performed only on the fixing eye.
Prism and cover are removed and the test is repeated with larger prisms.
The deviation is therefore measured using minimum dissociation until the point of reversal. The size of the manifest component is recorded as the prism value just before reversal of the eye movement.

Recording findings
25 alt XOT with 4 RhyperT-alternating heterotropia (prism bar used).

Expected findings
This depends on the size of any heterotropia and heterophoria present.

Chapter 10 Near point of convergence

Introduction
This is the point where visual axes intersect under maximum convergence effort while binocular single vision is maintained.

Use
The near point of convergence (NPC) is measured routinely, but especially when a patent presents with near vision symptoms, and can be carried out as a pre-refraction and post refraction test.

Procedure
Room lights on.
Appropriate near refractive correction should be worn.
Target may consist of a line target (RAF rule- our preferred method-see figure 8) or a pen tip held at 50 cm in front and slightly below midline of the patient (fine targets may cause confusion between blur and diplopia).
Illuminate target with local lighting if necessary.
Explain: This test determines how well your eyes converge to a close object.
Instruct: Please watch the object as I move it towards you and tell me if it goes double so that you see two objects instead of one.
For presbyopes, explain: The object may blur before it goes double.

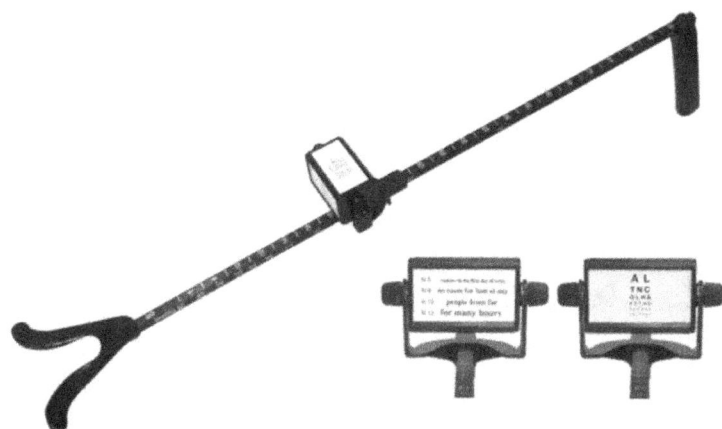

Figure 8 RAF rule with vertical line target for measuring NPC
Move target slowly towards bridge of nose (should take ~ 10s).
Measure the distance (cm) from target to bridge of nose
If/when patient reports diplopia (subjective break point).If/when one eye loses fixation (objective break point).

If diplopia reported then encourage patient to make single again (pull target back a little), then continue to move forward.
Check if reported diplopia is being confused with blur by covering one eye and asking whether diplopia still present.
After break point, slowly move target away until fixation/single vision restored (subjective/objective recovery point).
Measuring recovery point is not possible if NPC is to nose.

Recording findings
If break point never occurs then record 'NPC: to nose'.
Otherwise, record 'NPC: break point cm / recovery point cm'.
If subjective and objective measurements coincide (as is usual), no need to specify whether NPC is objective or subjective.

Hints and tips
Normal values: break ≤ 7.5 cm / recovery ≤ 10.5 cm.
Convergence insufficiency
Can cause fatigue and diplopia with prolonged close work.
Has high prevalence (up to 13% in older children).
Is easily treated (pencil push-up exercises).
Further investigations: jump convergence, fusional reserves.
Suspect suppression if objective break point occurs before subjective break point.
Record as: NPC: 14 cm / 18 cm, LE out, suppression?
May have to record objective NPC if diplopia confused with blur.
Record as NPC (Objective) 5 cm / 8 cm.

Chapter 11 Accommodative amplitude

Introduction
This is a measure of the maximum amount of accommodation an individual can exert. It can be described as the dioptric distance between the near and far points of accommodation and is usually measured using a RAF rule.

Use
It should be conducted monocularly and binocularly and may be repeated two or three times in those situations when patient symptoms are suggestive of accommodative fatigue.

Procedure
Keep room lights on.
Ask patient to wear their distance refractive correction (if appropriate).
Advise the patient: I am going to measure your focusing power.
Place RAF rule against patient's face with the prongs either side of the nose and the rule angled downwards at 45 degrees.
Make sure that the text block on the rule is well illuminated.
Ask patient to occlude the LE with a cover stick.
Instruct the patient to: look at the smallest print you can see. Advise the patient: I am going to move the print closer. Tell me when it first becomes blurred.
Push the text block slowly towards the patient.
When the patient reports that the print is blurred blur, ask them to: try and make it clear again.
Push the text block forward until the blur cannot be cleared; this gives the push-up amplitude.
Note this value in dioptres.
This can be read directly from the RAF rule.
Note, the RAF rule is also graduated in cm and orthoptists and ophthalmologists record accommodative amplitude using these units.
Push the text block further forward and then pull it slowly away from patient and ask: Tell me when it becomes clear again. This gives the pull-down amplitude of accommodation.
Note this value in dioptres.
The amplitude of accommodation is the average of the push up and pull down values.

Record findings
Amp (push-up/pull-down) RE 8D, LE 8D, BE 10D.

Expected findings
These will vary according to the age of the patient, see Table 1.

Monocular amplitude of accommodation and age based upon Duane-Hoffstetter formulae

Age	Minimum 15.0 − 0.25age	Average 18.5 − 0.30age	Maximum 25.0 − 0.40age
10	12.50	15.50	21.00
20	10.00	12.50	17.00
30	7.50	9.50	13.00
40	5.00	6.50	9.00
45	3.75	5.00	7.00
50	2.50	3.50	5.00
55	1.25	2.00	3.00
60	0.00	0.50	1.00

Note: these amplitudes include depth of focus

Table 1 Monocular amplitude of accommodation versus age.

Hints and tips
Children should be advised to read the smallest line they can resolve to themselves. The presence of saccadic eye movements would indicate that the child is attending to the task and will therefore be accommodating during the assessment, thus producing more accurate results.

Amplitude of accommodation can be artificially raised by depth of focus.

Size of letters increases as the text block is bought closer. Can instruct the patient to use smaller print as the text is moved closer. Can put -3.00DS lens in front of young patient's eyes so that near point is moved further away from eyes; 5D on the RAF rule then represents (3 + 5 =) 8D amplitude.

If the accommodative amplitude is >1.50DS lower than expected for age then accommodation insufficiency should be suspected.

Binocular amplitude should be ~ 1-2D greater than monocular amplitudes.

Chapter 12 Random dot stereograms

Introduction
The measurement of stereopsis is important as it gives an indication of the integrity of the binocular visual system. Stereopsis, also described as third degree fusion occurs when perceptual blending achieves the ultimate goal of depth perception based on retinal disparity. This can be demonstrated using stereotests.

Use
When the level of stereopsis (stereoacuity) is within expected ranges then normal motor and sensory function are present. It is particularly useful for evaluating binocular vision in children as obstacles to normal visual development early in life reduce the level of stereopsis attained and stereopsis is poor or absent in patients with heterotropia and amblyopia.

TNO

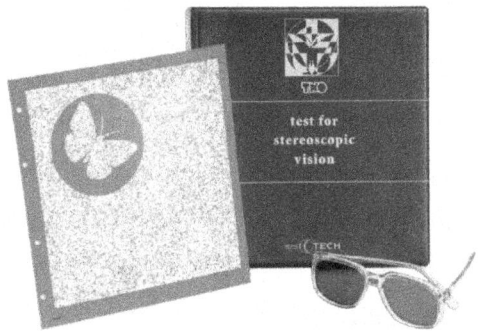

Figure 9 TNO stereopsis test.

Depth created by horizontal displacement of a group of elements in a random array (global stereopsis).
For children (4+ years) and adults.
Lacks monocular cues.
Our favoured test.
Room and local lights on.
Near correction worn if required.
Explain: I am now going to test your 3D vision.
Instruct: Please put these goggles on.
Red/green goggles worn (anaglyph test).
Red (LE), green (RE).
Wearing goggles may not be ideal for children aged <4 years.

Hold test at 40cm from patient.
Targets seen in crossed disparity (they appear to be in front of page).

Screening Plate I:
- Two butterflies
- One monocular (in a disc)
- One stereoscopic (hidden).
- Ask: How many butterflies can you see? And: Please point to them.

Two butterflies seen if gross stereopsis (1980 sec) is present.

Screening Plate II:
- Four circles:
- Two monocular
- Two stereoscopic (hidden)
- Ask: How many circles can you see? And: Point to the biggest one.
- Four seen if gross stereopsis (1980 sec) is present.

Screening Plate III:
- Four stereo shapes
- Central monocular cross
- Stereoscopic square, triangle, circle and diamond
- Ask: Can you find a cross/square/triangle/circle/diamond? And: Point to them.
- Four hidden shapes seen if gross stereopsis (1980 sec) is present.
- Advisable to just present this plate if the patient has a short attention span.

Screening Plate IV (this is a test for suppression and not stereoacuity):
- Three circles
- One mono RE (right circle)
- One mono LE (left circle)
- One binocular (centre).
- Ask: How many circles can you see? And: Point to them.
- Responses:
- Three seen = no suppression
- Two seen (right circle missing) = suppression right eye
- Two seen (left circle missing) = suppression left eye.

Measuring stereoacuity Plate V:
- Top two circles (480 sec)
- Bottom two circles (240 sec)
- Instruct/ask: In each of these squares there is a hidden cake with a piece missing. Can you find the cake and point to the piece that is missing?
- Measuring stereoacuity Plate VI:
- Top two circles (120 sec)
- Bottom two circles (60 sec)
- Instruct/ask: In each of these squares there is a hidden cake with a piece missing. Can you find the cake and point to the piece that is missing?

Measuring stereoacuity Plate VII:
- Top two circles (30 sec)
- Bottom two circles (15 sec)
- Instruct/ask: In each of these squares there is a hidden cake with a piece missing. Can you find the cake and point to the piece that is missing?

Hints and tips
Allow time to respond.
If only one of the two discs is described correctly then allow second attempt at incorrect one.
Record stereoacuity corresponding to last level for which both discs were correctly described.
When a patient fails one of plates V-VII return to one of the previous plates and ask them to 'find the cake and point to the piece that is missing'. They have already correctly identified the cake and where the piece is missing so should be able to do so again. This way the patient can finish the test on a positive note.

Recording findings
For plates V-VII, record stereoacuity as 'at least' ($\leq$) the highest level where both responses were correct.
If only plates I-III completed record 'TNO: gross stereopsis'.
If plate IV incorrect, record 'TNO: suppression RE/LE'.

Expected findings
At least 60 secs of stereoacuity to be considered within normal limits.

Chapter 13 Oculomotility

Introduction
It is useful to test oculomotility (smooth pursuit eye movements) for a whole range of reasons but in particular when a patient presents with diplopia, there are symptoms such as eye pain when looking away from the primary position of gaze and when there is a reading difficulty which is unlikely to be explained by the onset of presbyopia. Before oculomotility can be assessed accurately, good knowledge of the primary actions of the extraocular muscles is mandatory. See Figure 10 and Table 2.

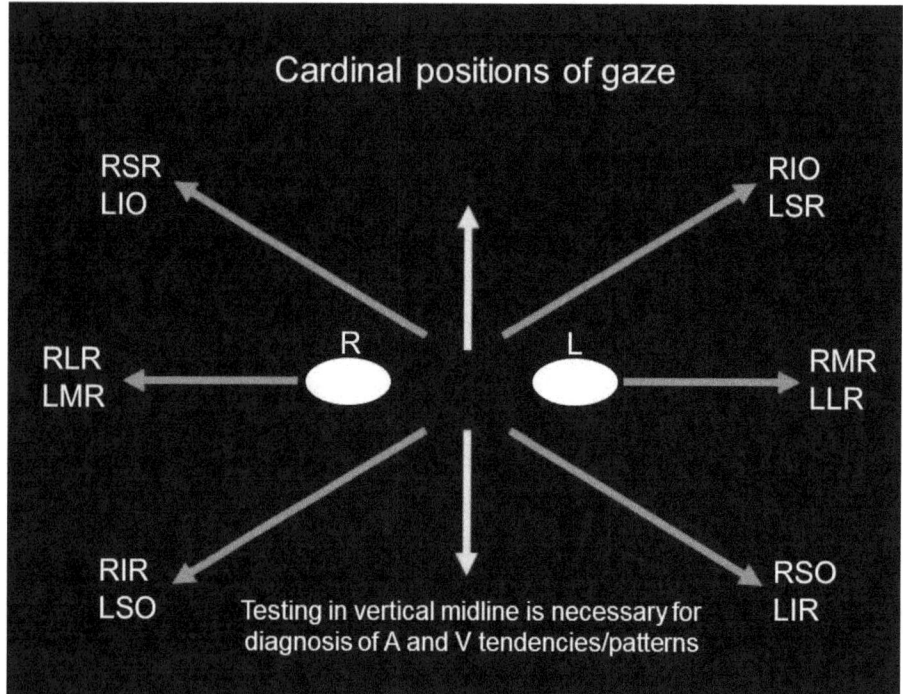

Figure 10 Cardinal positions of gaze.
RSR right superior rectus, RIO right inferior oblique, RMR right medial rectus, RSO RIR right inferior oblique, RLR right lateral rectus and the same for the left eye.

Duction	Agonist (this contracts)	Antagonist (this relaxes)
Abduction	LR	MR
Adduction	MR	LR
Supraduction	SR, IO	IR, SO
Infraduction	IR, SO	SR, IO
Incycloduction	SO, SR	IO, IR
Excycloduction	IO, IR	SO, SR

Table 2 Extra-ocular muscles involved with ductions.
LR, lateral rectus: MR, medial rectus; SR, superior rectus; IR, inferior rectus; SO, superior oblique; IO, inferior oblique.

Use
To elicit the extent and quality of movement of each eye.
To determine the presence of comitancy or incomitancy and whether any change in the size of the deviation is due to decompensation of a latent deviation or a muscle defect.
To establish the integrity of the ocular movement systems and their neural pathways.

Procedure
Use the spotlight from a pen torch held at 50 cm and sit directly in front of the patient so both eyes can be seen.
Always remove the patient's glasses for the following reasons:
Frames and the increase in effective power at the lens periphery limit the field of view.
Prismatic effects are induced in the lens periphery.
Reflection of spotlight on the lenses can confuse the interpretation of the findings.
Give clear instructions to the patient:
Keep the head straight and in the primary position throughout testing.
To report if at any point the patient appreciates diplopia (horizontal, vertical, torsional or a combination) and in which position it is maximum, or a change in diplopia if it is present in the primary position of gaze.
To report if any discomfort/pain during testing.
When in the primary position of gaze ask: Is the spotlight is double?
Move the spotlight slowly and smoothly from the primary position each time into the extremes of gaze, ensuring that the corneal reflections are present on each eye.
An audible/colourful fixation target may need to be used instead of or in combination with a spotlight for young children.
Perform the alternating cover test in the primary position comparing primary and secondary angles of deviation.

Test horizontal versions and look for the following:
- Up drift or down drift of either eye
- Underaction or overaction of movement
- Limitation (restriction of movement
- Changes in the size of the palpebral aperture
- Changes in pupil size

- Changes globe position.

Repeat the alternating cover test in the extreme positions of gaze. The size of the dissociated deviation will increase in the direction of the affected muscle(s).
If any defect is found on ductions and versions, (see Figure 11 for duction movements and Figure 12 for versions) it should be assessed, i.e. in the primary position occlude the fixing eye and observe the position of the corneal reflection as the spotlight is moved into the extreme position of gaze. There are two possible results:
The eye takes up fixation of the light, the corneal reflection remains central for the whole excursion and the movement is full. This indicates an under action of that muscle.
The eye takes up fixation for part of the excursion followed by cessation of movement and the corneal reflection is no longer central. This indicates a limitation (restriction) of movement.

Test direct elevation and observe for:
- Under action/over action/limitation
- Globe changes
- Simpson's test; check for signs of muscle fatigue by testing sustained elevation.
- When testing direct depression first perform without raising the upper lids so that any associated anomalies of lid movement can be seen.

Oblique positions; test elevated positions first to directly compare the same synergistic pairs of muscles in R and L gaze followed by the depressed positions and observe for:
- Underaction, overaction or limitation
- Changes in globe position
- Changes in lid position or lid movement.

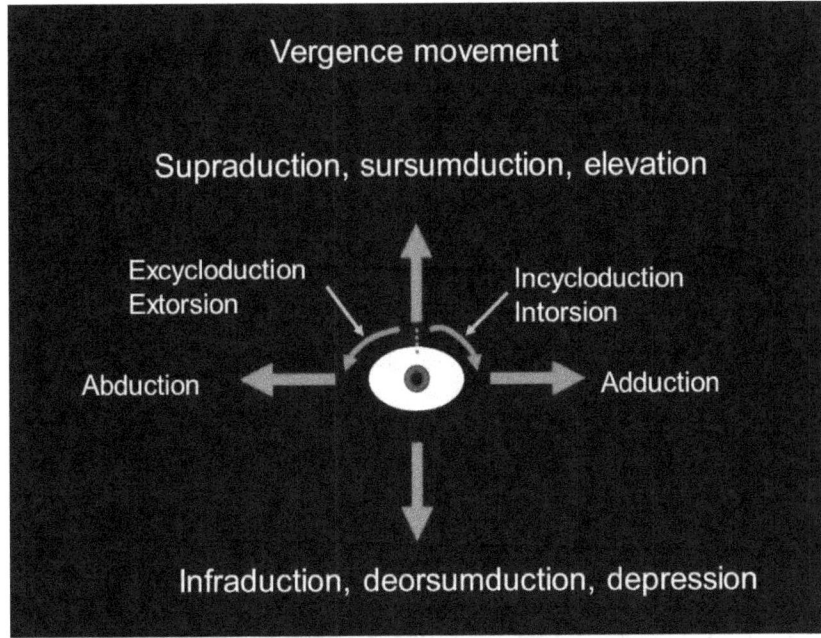

Figure 11 Duction movements of the right eye.

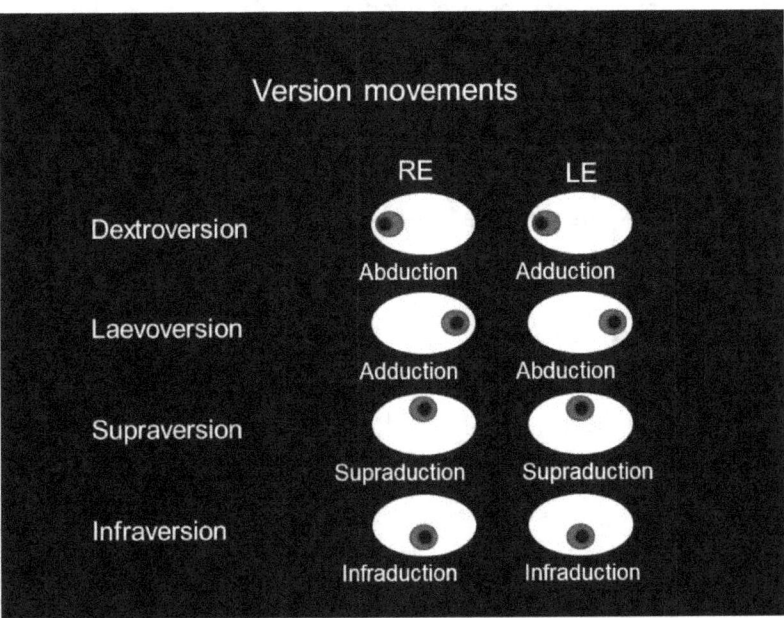

Figure 12 Classification of version movements.
Note, versions involve the movements of both eyes.

Hints and tips

The alternating cover test in direct elevation and depression is compared to elicit the presence of an A or V pattern i.e. a change in the horizontal angle of deviation (other patterns can exist e.g. Y or X).

Measured using the prism cover test an A pattern is diagnosed if there is a difference of ≥ 10Δ in eye position between the direct elevation and depression.
A V pattern is diagnosed if there is a difference of ≥ 15Δ (this takes into account the physiological V pattern of approximately 5Δ).
Patterns are due to imbalances between the vertically acting muscles, which produce horizontal changes from their secondary muscle actions.
Consider testing ductions during the initial oculo-motility test or by repeating the test.
Duction testing:
Discriminates between paretic and mechanical incomitancy.
If less under action occurs during duction than version movement then paresis is more likely.
If similar under action occurs during duction and version movement then mechanical restriction more likely.

Expected findings
SAFE-Smooth Accurate Full Extensive.

Recording findings
If no abnormality detected write SAFE (Smooth Accurate Full Extensive).

If abnormality detected, record the position of the eyes (use version terminology) in which:
- Patient reports diplopia or discomfort.
- Ask whether diplopia is horizontal or vertical.
- Diplopia is greatest (indicates direction of greatest under action).
- Cover each eye in turn to determine which sees the furthest image (the paretic eye carries the furthest image) or conduct alternating cover test in this position of gaze.
- Any under action or over action (record which eye) is detected.
- Jerky or inaccurate pursuit eye movements occur.

Chapter 14 Cover test with oculomotility in nine positions of gaze

Introduction
Follow the set-up procedure for oculomotility testing using a spotlight. Conduct an alternating cover test in the primary position of gaze.

Procedure
Repeat the alternate cover test in the extreme positions of gaze. The size of the dissociated deviation will increase in the direction of the affected muscle(s). If any defect is found on versions, ductions should be assessed, that is, in the primary position occlude the fixing eye and observe the position of the corneal reflection as the spotlight is moved into the extreme position of gaze.

There are two possible results:
- On occlusion of the fixing eye, the suspect eye takes up fixation of the light, the corneal reflection remains central for the whole excursion and the movement is full-this indicates an under action of the muscle that acts maximally in this position of gaze.
- On occlusion of the fixing eye, the suspect eye takes up fixation for part of the excursion followed by cessation of movement and the corneal reflection is no longer central-this indicates a limitation (restriction) of movement.

Test direct elevation and observe for:
- Underaction, overaction and limitation
- Globe changes
- Signs of lid or extraocular muscle fatigue by testing sustained elevation (Simpson's test).

Hints and tips
When testing direct depression, first perform without raising the upper lids so that any associated anomalies of lid movement can be seen.

Expected findings
SAFE- Smooth Accurate Full Extensive.

Recording findings
If no abnormality detected, write SAFE.

If abnormality is detected, record the position of the eyes (use version terminology) in which:

- Patient reports diplopia or discomfort.
- Ask whether diplopia is horizontal or vertical.
- Diplopia is greatest (indicates direction of greatest underaction).
- Cover each eye in turn to determine which sees the furthest image (the paretic eye carries the furthest image) or conduct alternating cover test in this position of gaze.
- Any underaction or overaction (record which eye) is directed.
- Jerky or inaccurate smooth pursuit eye movements occur.

Chapter 15 Interpupillary distance

Introduction
This measurement can be taken at any time during pre-refraction but is often conducted just before the trial frame is placed on the patient's face. It is a quick and simple procedure in the hands of a reasonably skilled practitioner but is often undertaken incorrectly by novices and those that rush.

Use
To set up the trial frame correctly.
To order lenses with the correct optical centres during the dispensing process.
To be able to determine if there is any prism incorporated into the current lenses (if there are any current spectacles) by comparing the measured interpupillary distance with the optical centres of the current lenses.

Procedure
1. For the distance viewing interpupillary distance, sit at approximately arm's length and directly in front of the patient.
2. At arm's length place a PD rule across the patients brow so that the '0 mm' (zero) mark on the ruler scale is approximately in line with the temporal pupil margin of the patient's right eye.
3. Close your right eye, and looking only with your left eye adjust the alignment (if required) of the PD rule's zero to the temporal pupil margin of the patient's right eye.
4. Without moving the ruler, open your left eye close your right eye.
5. Look at the nasal pupil margin of the patient's left eye and note the value on the PD rule to the nearest millimetre.
6. Remember this value as the interpupillary distance (for distance viewing) in millimetres.
7. For the near interpupillary distance, keep the ruler in place on the patient's brow, open both of your eyes and move one of your index fingers so it is in the patient's primary position of gaze and around 33 cm from the patient.
8. Adjust the PD rules zero mark so it is in line with the right eye temporal pupil margin and with both of your eyes open and look at the left eye nasal pupil margin and note the value on the PD rule to the nearest millimetre.
9. Note the distance and near interpupillary distances in the clinical records.

Hints and tips
Some practitioners will, instead of measuring the near interpupillary distance, simply subtract 3 mm from the distance viewing interpupillary distance.
Our view is that as it only takes a few seconds to accurately measure the near interpupillary distance, it is better to actually measure it rather than estimate it.

Recording findings
PD 66/63; the first number is the distance viewing interpupillary distance and the second the near interpupillary distance.

IPD 63/59.

Expected findings
For a man, values of around 66/63 would be expected with less for a woman (as women are often smaller than men) for example, 63/59.

Chapter 16 Trial frame set up

Introduction
Accurate trial frame set-up is essential to determine optimum refractive correction, visual acuity, reading acuity and other potential post-refraction values such as aligning prism.

Use
To hold and adjust spherical and cylindrical trial lenses during retinoscopy.
To hold and adjust spherical and cylindrical trial lenses during subjective refraction.
To hold prism lenses during aligning prism determination.
To measure distance visual acuity and near reading acuity.

Procedure
Right and left monocular pupillary distances can be adjusted by rotating the adjusting knob of each eye, located above each lens well. The arrows above the lens wells indicate each monocular pupillary distance. Adding the PD values for each eye equals the binocular PD value.
The temple length can be adjusted by loosening the knob on top of the temple and pulling on the end of the temple. When the correct temple length has been established, the knob may be tightened to secure the length.
There are two knobs that control the position of the nose pad. The knob at the top of the frame controls the height of the nose pad. The angle of the frame in relation to the patient's face is controlled by the knob on the front of the frame. When adjusting the nose pad, remember that the standard distance from the lens to the cornea is 12mm.
Centre the patient's eyes with the optical centres of the lenses.
For optimal optical clarity, insert the least number of lenses possible to create the desired power.
The highest powered lens should be placed closest to the cornea (in the back lens clamp/cell).
Always replace the trial lenses in the case when not in use.
Insert the lens quickly and accurately.

Hints and tips
Make sure your temple is slightly angled up so that there is a pantoscopic tilt of around 10 degrees. This mimics the recommended pantoscopic tilt for spectacle frames.
Adjust the temple to fit snuggly behind the ear making sure the patient is as comfortable as can be expected while wearing a trial frame.
Ensure the frame is straight.

Check the pupillary distance of the trial frame matches the pupillary distance of the patient.
Ensure the nose rest is up on the nose.
Check that the patient is looking through the centre of the lens(s).

SECTION 2 REFRACTION

Chapter 17 Spot retinoscopy

Chapter 18 Near fixation retinoscopy (Mohindra technique)

Chapter 19 Jackson cross cylinder (JCC)

Chapter 20 Binocular balancing

Chapter 21 Binocular addition

Chapter 22 Determination of the near add

Chapter 17 Spot retinoscopy

Introduction
Retinoscopy is an objective technique for determination of refractive error.

Use
Retinoscopy can provide a good approximation of refractive error and this is particularly useful in cases where the patient finds it difficult to communicate, new patients who have not brought their glasses to the consultation and those who have not had a refractive correction in the past. In these cases the power of the trial lenses determined through retinoscopy provide a useful starting point for subjective refraction.

Procedure
Put a trial frame on the patient and set the distance pupillary distance.
Switch on the duochrome and explain the test: I'm going to shine a light in your eye to find out whether you need glasses. Please look at the green target and let me know if my head blocks your view. Don't worry if the target is blurred. The green target less likely to stimulate accommodation in young patients
Turn the room lights off.
Sit in front of the patient on their right hand side and use your right eye for retinoscopy:
Use a working distance of 67 cm when possible.
Push retinoscope collar down for maximum beam divergence.
Relax accommodation in patient's fixating left by placing increasing plus lenses in the left cell of the trial frame until the retinoscopy reflex (also known as ret reflex) has against movements in all meridians:
This is not necessary if the patient already displays an against movement of the retinoscope reflex, that is, they are myopic or they are over 60 years old and have no amplitude of accommodation.
With the patient looking at the green duochrome target observe the reflex in orthogonal (180°/90°) and oblique (45°/135°) meridians.
Neutralise the ret reflex in the right eye using spherical and if necessary cylindrical lenses:
View along the visual axis of the right eye and make sure the patient can always see the green duochrome fixation target.
Always place spherical lenses in the rear cell of the trial frame to keep the back vertex distance to a minimum and reduce errors due to effectivity.
When there is astigmatic refractive error, with the streak retinoscope rotate the streak until it coincides with the angle of the reflex movement:
This will occur in two mutually perpendicular meridians.

With the spot retinoscope the ret reflex will appear elliptical with its major and minor axes aligned to both astigmatic meridians.
Neutralise most plus/least minus meridian.
Slowest 'with' ret reflex movement if both meridians are plus.
Fastest 'against' ret reflex movement if both meridians are minus.
Move the retinoscope beam along the meridian e.g. horizontal meridian neutralised by moving the beam (spot or vertical streak) horizontally.
Use bracketing to neutralise the reflex.
Now check neutral point by moving slightly forward ('with' movement) and backwards ('against' movement).
Neutralise second meridian (perpendicular to first).
An 'against' reflex should be seen:
If not, simply add plus to neutralise 'with' movement.
Then return to first meridian that will be 'against'.
Set minus cylinder axis perpendicular to second meridian (i.e. parallel to streak).
Use bracketing to neutralise reflex.
Moving collar up can help when close to neutral as it makes reflex easier to see.
REMEMBER to add minus cylinder to neutralise 'with' movement when collar is up.
Check sphere and cylinder:
Move slightly forward (equal 'with' in both meridians).
Move slightly backward (equal 'against' in both meridians).
Check cylinder axis:
Compare reflex when ret beam is moved 45° either side of the cylinder axis.
If cylinder axis incorrect, one reflex will be 'with' and the other 'against'.
Rotate the trial cylinder axis in the direction of the ret beam that produces the 'with' reflex.
Both reflexes will be the same when the trial cylinder axis is correct
Move across to the patient's left hand side and remove any trial lens used to relax accommodation from in front of the LE.
Repeat procedure for LE.
Measure VA of R and LE.

Recording findings
Subtract 1.50DS to take into account the 67 cm working distance.
Note power of trial lenses remaining in the trial frame after the working distance allowance has been made.
When recording the results:
Write clearly.
Avoid using the degree sign (°) for cylinder axis as this may be confused with 0.
Record sphere and cyl power to nearest 0.25D.
Record cylinder axis to nearest 2.5.
Cylinder axis should be between 2.5 and 180 – not 0.

Hints and tips
When the ret reflex is dim or slow moving then add lenses to get closer to neutral.
The brighter, faster and wider the ret reflex is the closer is the neutral point.
When ret reflex movement is the same in all meridians then the refractive error is very likely to be spherical.

When ret reflex movement differs in each meridian then the refractive error will have an astigmatic component.

Common errors are:
- Incorrect working distance or collar position
- Spherical errors
- Working off axis
- Astigmatic errors
- Oblique astigmatism tends to be against the rule
- Blocking patient's view of the chart
- Stimulates accommodation
- Spherical errors (under-plus, over-minus)
- Not concentrating on centre of reflex with large pupils
- Spherical aberration, more 'against' reflex in periphery
- Spherical errors (under-plus, over-minus)
- Ret result is often more plus than subjective
- Most evident in young
- Least evident in presbyope.

Chapter 18 Near fixation retinoscopy (Mohindra technique)

Introduction
There are some potential adverse reactions, side effects and legal issues on the use of cycloplegic drugs. Alternatives to using drugs have been suggested. One such method is near fixation retinoscopy, often referred to as the Mohindra technique. This relies on the fact that young children are likely to be attracted to a retinoscope light in a darkened room. To keep the infant attentive it has been suggested that feeding them can help; feeding also helps to relax the accommodation and widens the palpebral aperture.

Use
Noncycloplegic retinoscopy can be used when frequent follow up is necessary, when the child is extremely anxious about instillation of cycloplegic agents and when the child has had or is at risk of an adverse reaction to cycloplegic drugs.

Procedure
Retinoscopy is carried out in a totally dark room at 50 cm on one eye while the examiner or a carer occludes the other eye.
It is assumed that the eye undergoing retinoscopy is at its resting accommodation level when the retinoscopy light is maintained at a minimum.
Retinoscopy is performed by neutralising the retinal reflex in the two primary meridians of the eye using loose trial lenses.
The gross sphere cylinder form is then calculated from the meridional findings.
Results from a study of infant subjects indicated greater agreement between near and cycloplegic retinoscopy (two drops of 1% cyclopentolate) when 1.00 DS is subtracted from the spherical component of the gross retinoscopy result for those patients less than two years of age, and 0.75 DS subtracted for those over the age of two years.
These values allow for the 50 cm working distance and tonus.

Opinions vary as to the accuracy of this technique. If during retinoscopy, the light does not provide a stimulus to accommodation and the eye assumes its normal resting state of accommodation it would seem that the results from this technique would be reasonably reliable. However, it has been proposed that tonus is dependent on the type of refractive error present, with hyperopes having a greater amount. If this were true then it would result in the Mohindra technique underestimating the amount of hyperopia seen.

Hints and tips
Make sure that the room is dark.
Remember to occlude the eye not being refracted.
Many practitioners use a refraction 'cross' to record the power of the spherical lenses required to reduce each meridian.

Recording findings

Example 1: A three-year-old patient.

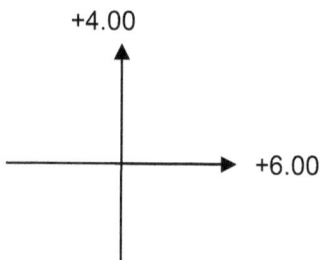

Raw result +4.00/+2.00 x 90

Tonus and working distance allowance -1.00

Final result +3.00/+2.00 x 90

Example 2: A one-year-old patient.

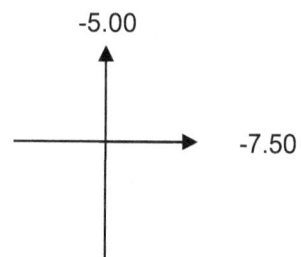

Raw result -7.50/+2.50 x 180

Tonus and working distance allowance -0.75

Final result -7.75/+2.50 x 180

Example 3: A four-year-old patient.

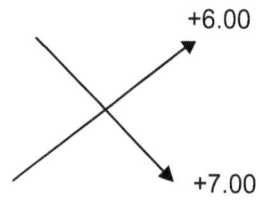

Raw result +6.00/+1.00 x 45

Tonus and working distance allowance -1.00

Final result +5.00/+1.00 x 45

Chapter 19 Jackson cross cylinder (JCC)

Introduction
Although retinoscopy provides a reasonable approximation of refractive correction because of errors arising from working off the visual axis and spherical aberration, before a prescription can be issued the results obtained need to be refined during subjective refraction.

Use
Subjective refraction involves a series of procedures that enable the accurate determination of distance and near refractive correction.

Procedure
Refining the sphere for best VA
Begin with the sphere or sphere-cylinder in place found during static retinoscopy (working distance lens removed).
Turn room lights on and explain: During this test, I will place various lenses in front of your eye to find those that give you the best vision. Don't worry about giving a wrong answer as everything is double checked.
Test right eye first and occlude the left eye.
Switch on the letter chart and ask: Please look at the smallest line you can see.
Add +0.25DS and ask: Are the letters clearer, more blurred or the same?
If clearer or the same, keep adding +0.25DS lenses until letters on the smallest line the patient could see blur.
This will give the sphere for best VA.
If when adding +0.25DS the letters on the smallest line become blurred, don't add +0.25DS but proceed to next step.
Add -0.25DS and ask: Are the letters clearer now or just smaller and blacker?
If clearer, keep adding -0.25DS lenses until no further improvement in the sharpness of the letters on the smallest line occurs.
This will give the sphere for best VA.
If the letters become smaller and blacker but not sharper, don't add -0.25DS. The sphere for best VA will have been found.

Refining the cyl axis using the Jackson Cross Cyl (JCC)
Add -0.25DS to sphere in young patients.
Select JCC: ±0.25DC for a starting VA 6/12 or better, ±0.50DC for starting VA 6/18 or worse.
Illuminate on the concentric ring or cluster dot target and ask: I want you to compare the clarity of the rings (dots) while I hold this lens in two positions. The rings (dots) may look slightly blurred in both positions but tell me which position is clearer or whether they both look the same.

Flip JCC with its handle along the trial cyl axis and ask: Clearer in position 1 or 2.
Move the trial cyl axis towards the minus cyl axis of the preferred JCC position.
Continue, using '3 or 4', '4 or 5' … until no difference can be detected by the patient when viewing the rings (or dots).
If no cyl was found during retinoscopy, check JCC at axes 90/180 and 45/135.

Refining the cyl power using the JCC
Position the JCC with one of its axes parallel to the trial cyl axis and ask: Clearer in position 1 or 2.
Increase cyl power if minus JCC axis preferred.
Reduce cyl power if plus JCC axis preferred.
Vice versa if working in positive cyl during retinoscopy.
Continue, using '3 or 4', '4 or 5' … until no difference detected.
Add +0.25DS to the trial lens sphere for every -0.50DC increase in cyl power (and *vice versa*).
If significant change to trial cyl power or axis, re-check sphere to achieve best VA.
Measure monocular VA.
If VA improves with pinhole then re-check subjective refraction.
Check test:
+1.00DS trial lens placed in front of each eye monocularly should reduce VA to ~ 6/18.
Repeat JCC on the LE with the RE occluded.

Recording findings
Note power of trial lenses in the trial frame after when subjective refraction is completed for each eye.

When recording result:
- Write clearly.
- Avoid using the degree sign (°) for cylinder axis as this may be confused with 0.
- Record sphere and cyl power to nearest 0.25D.
- Record cylinder axis to nearest 2.5.
- Cylinder axis should be between 2.5 and 180 – not 0.

Hints and tips
For those patients who find it difficult to understand what is required during cyl axis and power refinement using the JCC initially rotate the trial cyl axis 5-10° away from that found during retinoscopy so that a definite preference occurs and test is better understood.
The ±0.25DC JCC has a sphero-cyl power of +0.25/-0.50 and the ±0.50DC JCC a sphero-cyl power of +0.50/-1.00 (in the minus cyl form).
This is why when a patient accepts more minus or plus cyl power twice consecutively during refinement with the JCC the cyl power should be changed by 0.50DC and the sphere changed by 0.25DS.

Binocular refraction
Advantages
Accommodation remains balanced/relaxed throughout subjective refraction.
Good for hyperopia, pseudomyopia, antimetropia.
Avoids the need for occlusion.
Occlusion dilates the pupil and may lead to refractive changes due to spherical aberration.
Occlusion manifests latent nystagmus and can make subjective refraction difficult.
Occlusion manifests cyclophoria and can lead to incorrect assessment of astigmatism.
Takes less time than monocular refraction as no need for binocular balancing.

Disadvantages
Difficult for some patients with highly dominant eyes.
Poor subjective responses in non-dominant eye as patient will always be more aware of vision in dominant eye even if it is fogged.
It is better to refract these patients monocularly but there will still be problems with binocular balancing tests that involve using monocular fogging.

Methods
Monocular fogging.
Preferred technique.
Polarised refraction procedure.
Polarising filters reduce letter contrast making the test difficult for patients with cataract.
Turville infinite balance (TIB).
Cumbersome as it requires a septum.

Monocular fogging
Carry out static retinoscopy on each eye.
Fog LE with +0.75DS and check is VA 6/12.
Carry out JCC subjective refraction on RE.
Repeat procedure for LE while RE fogged.
Carry out binocular addition, if necessary.

There is no need for binocular balancing.

Chapter 20 Binocular balancing

Introduction
Following retinoscopy and subjective refraction, binocular balancing is used to ensure that the accommodation is balanced. It corrects any extra hyperopia that may become manifest when the patient becomes binocular.

Use
Binocular balancing ensures that accommodation is balanced between the two eyes as an imbalance often leads to asthenopia. Binocular balancing is not required if the patient is:
- Monocular
- Over 60 years of age
- Pseudophakic.

There are several techniques available:
- Monocular fogging (modified Humphriss)
  - Preferred technique (with trial frame)
- Prism-dissociated blur balance
  - Preferred if using phoropter/projected chart
- Humphriss immediate contrast (HIC)
  - Uses the effects of binocular summation and inhibition
- Turville infinite balance
  - Cumbersome as it requires a septum.

Monocular fogging
Accommodation is balanced and relaxed when using both eyes together. Under these conditions, the 'sphere for best VA' for each eye is determined. This is achieved by fogging one eye and testing the other. Fogging one eye suppresses central vision but maintains peripheral fusion so that both eyes work together (accommodation balanced/relaxed) and the 'sphere for best VA' can be found in the other eye

Procedure
Carry out static retinoscopy and monocular subjective refraction on both eyes.
Explain: I now want to see how well your eyes work together but this test requires the vision in one eye to be blurred.
Fog LE with +0.75DS.
Occlude the RE and ask: Although your vision is now blurred, please read the smallest line you can see.

VA should be about 6/12, add extra plus if not.
Remove occluder from RE and ask: please look at the smallest line you can see.
Add +0.25DS and ask: Are the letters clearer, more blurred or the same?
If clearer or the same, keep adding +0.25DS lenses until acuity first blurs; this is the sphere for best VA.
If blurred, don't add +0.25DS but proceed to next step.
Add -0.25DS and ask: Are the letters clearer now or just smaller and blacker?
If clearer, keep adding -0.25DS lenses until no further improvement in acuity occurs; this is the sphere for best VA.
If smaller and blacker, don't add -0.25DS.
Repeat the procedure with RE fogged.
Determine 'sphere for best VA' in LE.

Recording findings
Binocular balancing RE +0.25DS LE +0.50DS.

Expected findings
This depends on how well accommodation was controlled during subjective refraction.

Chapter 21 Binocular addition

Introduction
Accommodation relaxes in binocular single vision and therefore binocular addition may not be necessary as balancing with monocular fogging may have already relaxed accommodation maximally. However, this technique can be used as a final check to ensure that the accommodation is completely relaxed.

Use
Binocular addition can be useful for patients requiring maximum plus such as low hyperopes with near work symptoms. Note: some patients prefer under-plus or over-minus distance correction for everyday tasks especially driving. Remember that a 6m chart is at a dioptric distance of -0.16DS.

Procedure
Remove fogging lens used during binocular balancing so the patient can see clearly through both eyes.
Ask: Please look at the smallest line of letters you can see.
Add +0.25DS to both eyes and ask: Are the letters clearer, more blurred or the same?
If clearer or the same, keep adding +0.25DS lenses until acuity first blurs; the endpoint has been reached.
If more blurred, do not add +0.25DS.

Hints and tips
If the difference between retinoscopy and subjective prescription indicates latent hyperopia, an alternative method would be to add +1.00DS to both eyes and reduce in 0.25DS steps until best VA attained.

Recording findings
Binocular addition +0.25DS.

Expected findings
This depends on how well accommodation was controlled during subjective refraction.

Chapter 22 Determination of the near addition

Introduction
Presbyopia is a refractive condition in which the accommodative ability of the eye is insufficient for near vision work. It usually occurs at 40-45 years of age but may be earlier in people living in hot climates, people with short arms/working distances and hyperopes and later in people with long arms/working distances and myopes. The amplitude of accommodation falls to zero at about 55 years of age. After that age, the clinically measured amplitude of accommodation is likely to be due to depth of focus. Presbyopes need a near addition (plus lens addition to their distance prescription) that increases as they get older. The tentative add can be determined using:

- Age and working distance.
- Simplest, quickest and least prone to error.
- Amplitude of accommodation.
- Prone to error.
- Negative and positive relative accommodation.
- Even more error prone than using the amplitude of accommodation.
- Binocular cross-cylinder.
- Most error prone.

After the tentative add has been found the final add can be determined subjectively along with the range of clear near vision.

Determining the tentative add using age and working distance
Determine working distance needs from history and symptoms.
Reading distances may range from 33 to 40 cm.
Computer screens are often read from 50 to 60 cm.
Distances of less than 33cm may be required.
Hobbies (e.g. sewing)
Medicine bottles.

WD▶ Age▼	33 cm	40 cm	50-60 cm
45y	1.25	0.75	0.50
50y	1.75	1.25	1.00
55y	2.25	1.75	1.50
≥60y	2.50	2.00	1.75

Table 3 Tentative add based on the patients age and required working distance.

Determining the tentative add using amplitude of accommodation
Add = required working distance in dioptres - ½ amplitude of accommodation in dioptres.

For example,

Patient aged 50 years
Amplitude of accommodation = 3.50D
Required working distance is 33cm = 3.00D
Tentative add = 3.00 - ½(3.50) = 1.25D.

Determining the final add
Room lights on.
Only use extra illumination (e.g. a local lamp directed over patient's shoulder) if a reading light is normally used.
Explain: I am now going to determine the power of lens you need for reading.
Adjust trial frame for near PD.
Insert tentative add with distance correction in trial frame.
Give the patient the reading chart and instruct: Please hold the chart at your normal reading distance and look at the smallest letters that you can see.
Add -0.25DS lenses (use ±0.25DS flippers) binocularly and ask: Are the letters clearer, more blurred or the same?.
If clearer, continue adding -0.25DS lenses to both eyes until clarity does not improve; this gives the final add.
If more blurred don't add -0.25DS but proceed to next step.
Add +0.25DS and ask 'Are the letters clearer, more blurred or the same?.
If clearer, continue adding +0.25DS lenses to both eyes until clarity does not improve; this gives the final add.
If the same or more blurred, don't add +0.25DS; this gives the final add.

Art of Clinical Practice in Optometry

This ensures that you give most minus/least plus.
Record N-number of smallest letters read for RE, LE and for both eyes together.

Determining the range of clear vision

For example,

Patient aged 50 years.
Amplitude of accommodation = 3.50D.
Near add = 2.25D for a required working distance of 33cm.
Closest point of range = 1 ÷ (near add + amp).
i.e. patient uses total accommodative amplitude through near add.
Near point = 1 ÷ (2.25 + 3.50) = 0.17m or 17cm.
Farthest point of range = 1 ÷ (near add).
i.e. patient relaxes through near add.
Far point = 1 ÷ 2.25 = 0.44m or 44cm.
Maximum range of clear vision = 17 to 44cm.

Procedure
Explain: I will now demonstrate the range of distances over which these reading lenses work.
Ask: Please move the chart slowly towards you until the smallest letters you can see first become blurred.
Measure distance in cm; this gives the closest point of range
Ask: Now move the chart slowly away from you until the smallest letters you can see become blurred.
Measure distance in cm; this gives the farthest point of range
Ask: Are you happy with the range of distances that these lenses allow you to work at?
If yes, do not adjust final add.
If no, alter final add binocularly until the patient's needs are met.
Alternatively, provide an intermediate add.

Recording findings
Record the power of add for RE and LE along with the near word or letter acuity and the working range in cm.

Example, for reading   R +2.25 L+2.25 Range 17 to 44 cm   RVA N5 LVA N5 at 40 cm.

Example, for VDU use   R +1.50 L+1.50 Range 20 to 67 cm   RVA N5 LVA N5 at 55 cm.

Hints and tips
Near visual adequacy may be the only routine assessment of near vision carried out on pre-presbyopes.
Amplitudes of accommodation (and other accommodation tests) are only carried out if there are near vision symptoms.

Do not measure amplitudes of accommodation in patients aged over 55 years.
Near additions are usually equal in both eyes.
Adds rarely exceed +3.00DS but may do for some patients with low vision.

SECTION 3 POST REFRACTION

Chapter 23 Maddox rod

Chapter 24 Maddox wing

Chapter 25 Distance and near Mallett Unit

Chapter 26 Direct ophthalmoscopy-anterior segment examination

Chapter 27 Direct ophthalmoscopy-posterior segment examination

Chapter 28 External and anterior eye examination using direct illumination

Chapter 23 Maddox rod

Introduction
The Maddox rod (MR - distance and near) is used to quantify heterophoria and are particularly useful for the detection of small vertical heterophoria (<3 prism diopters - Δ) as these may be missed during the cover test, especially by the novice, and yet can still cause troublesome visual symptoms. It is often described as a dissociated or dissociating test as it disrupts fusion throughout the entire test so that both eyes move to their passive positions. During the cover test, dissociation only occurs while one eye is covered and only that eye moves to the passive position. Dissociating tests are indicated when:

- Cover test reveals large heterophoria.
- Cover test suggests that heterophoria uncompensated, e.g. slow recovery to pre-dissociation position.
- Refractive error has changed.

It is common for the cover test to be carried out pre-refraction with the patient wearing their glasses if they use them and subjective measures of heterophoria are performed post-refraction with the patient wearing a trial frame and correcting trial lenses. However, those practitioners that use a phoropter may prefer to use subjective measurements of heterophoria pre-refraction with the patient's current prescription dialled in and also post-refraction with the new prescription in place.

The MR does not give any information on the presence of a heterotropia and should only be used on patients with some level of binocularity.

The MR is a distortion test i.e. image presented to one eye is distorted to a level were fusion cannot occur. This distortion is produced by grooves (plano-convex cylinders) ground onto disc of coloured glass – red glass used for distance (see Figure 13) and green glass can be used for near. A spotlight seen through the disc is distorted into a streak of light at right angles to axis of grooves.

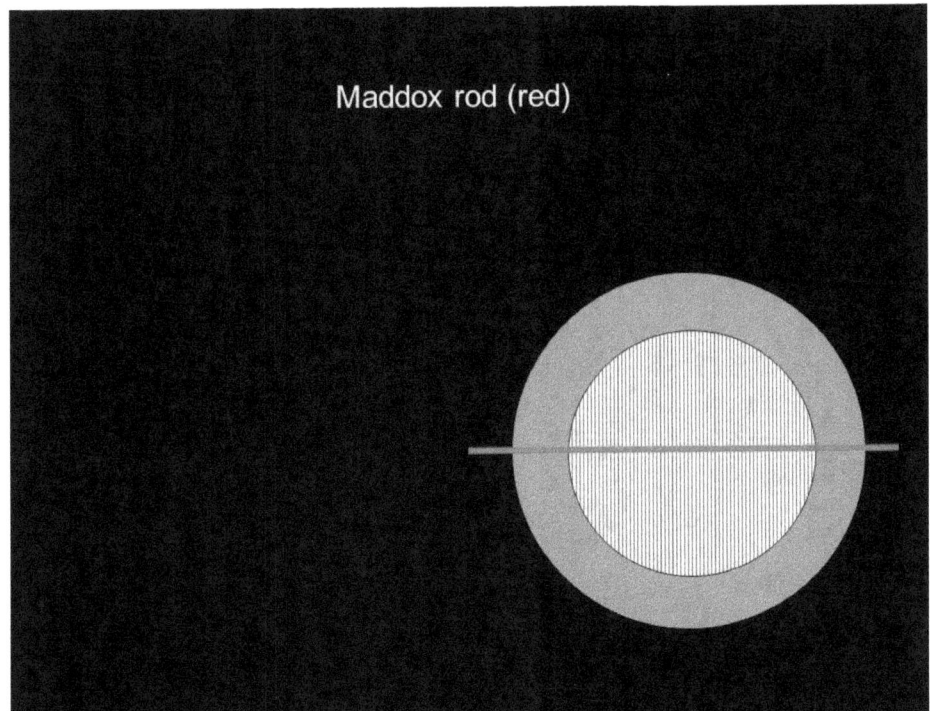

Figure 13 Maddox rod: red line seen by patient when grooves are vertical.

Use
The MR test is commonly only performed at distance with the Maddox wing being used for the assessment of heterophoria at near. It is mainly used for quantifying distance heterophoria.

Procedure
Explain: This test checks how well your eye muscles work together when looking in the distance.
Patient should wear appropriate refractive correction with correct distance papillary distance.
Place MR in front of the right eye, with grooves horizontal ready to test for horizontal phoria.
Room lights should be dimmed with a distance spotlight.
Ask: Please look at the chart. Can you see a spot light and a vertical red line?
Encourage patient to become aware of both targets by covering each eye in turn.
If the red line does not pass through the centre of the spot light then add appropriate prisms to left eye until the line passes through the spot. See Figure 14.
Repeat with MR grooves vertical to test for vertical phoria and ask: Is the horizontal red line above, below or straight through the spot? See Figure 15.

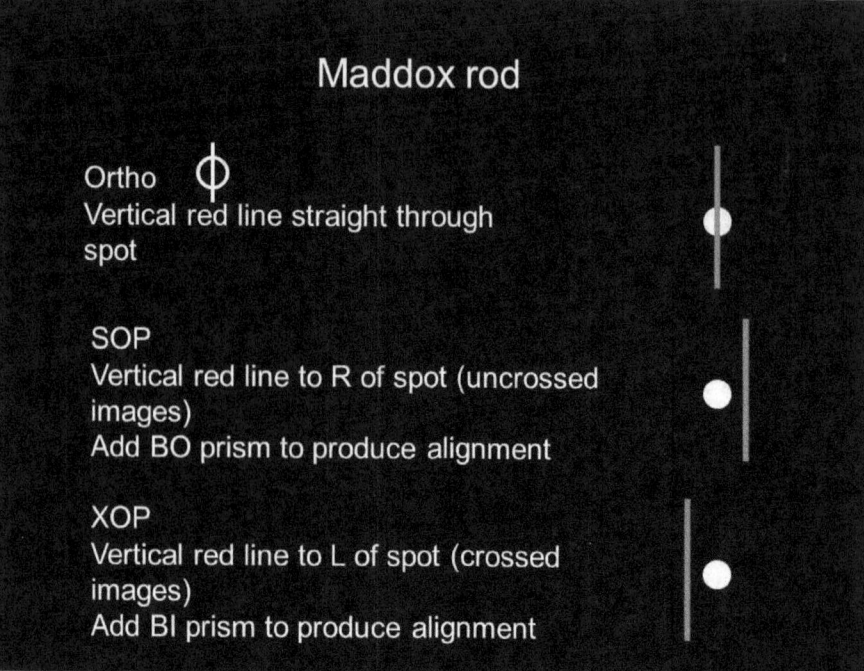

Figure 14 Add appropriate prisms to left eye until line passes through the spot.

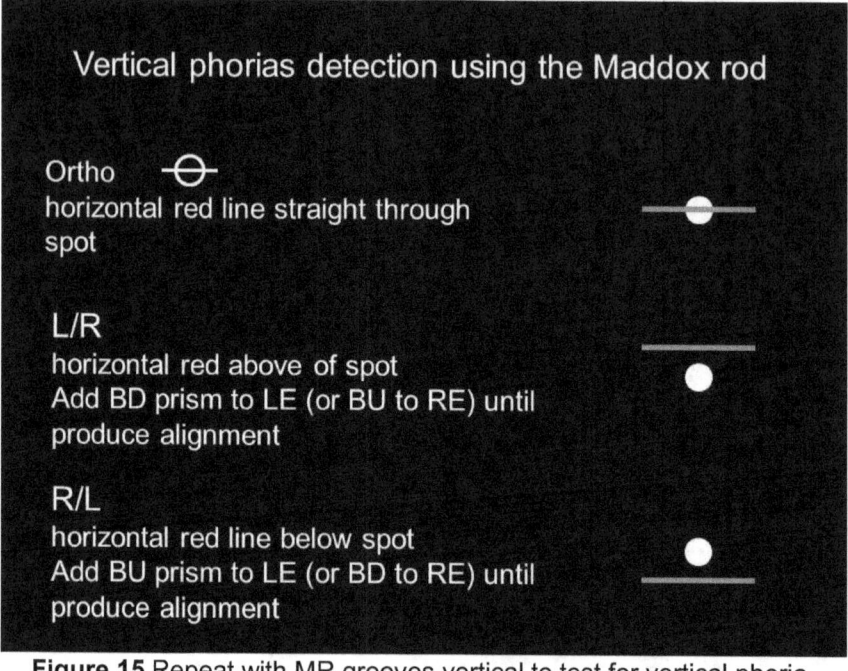

Figure 15 Repeat with MR grooves vertical to test for vertical phoria.

Double MR test
Grooves adjusted so vertical.
Green MR before LE.
Red MR before RE.
Ask patient to look at spot light on chart.
Vertically dissociate both eyes with prisms.
LE - 3Δ base-down, green MR.
RE - 3Δ base up, red MR.
Ask patient to rotate MRs in trial frame until images appear parallel.
This will give the angle of cyclophoria in degrees. See Figure 16.

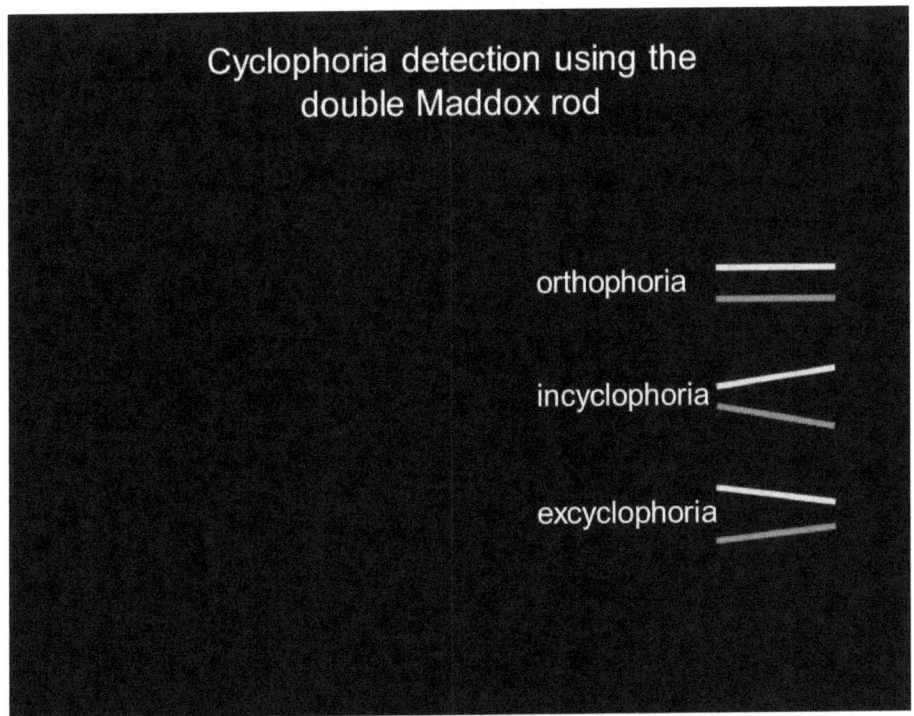

Figure 16 Detecting and measuring cyclophoria.

Hints and tips
Spotlight is poor stimulus for accommodation and therefore.
Exophoria is overestimated and esophoria underestimated.
Still useful for vertical and cyclophoria.
Arguably useful for patients over 55 years of age.

Most common errors:
- Allowing patient to adopt CHP.
- Assessing phoria in patient without any binocularity.
- Incorrect pupillary distance in trial frame.

Recording findings

MR – record the test carried out

──── horizontal and vertical orthophoria

1 R/L – horizontal orthophoria, 1$^\Delta$ R hyperphoria

3 SOP 3$^\Delta$ esophoria with vertical orthophoria

3 SOP 1 R/L – 3$^\Delta$ esophoria with 1$^\Delta$ R hyperphoria

RE suppression – test not carried out

Chapter 24 Maddox wing

Introduction
The Maddox wing (MW - near) is used to quantify heterophoria and is particularly useful for the detection of small vertical heterophoria (<3 Δ - Δ) as these may be missed during the cover test, especially by the novice, and yet can still cause troublesome visual symptoms. It is often described as a dissociated or dissociating test as it disrupts fusion throughout the entire test so that both eyes move to their passive positions. During the cover test, dissociation only occurs while one eye is covered and only that eye moves to the passive position. Dissociating tests are indicated when:

- Cover test reveals large heterophoria.
- Cover test suggests that heterophoria uncompensated, e.g. slow recovery to pre-dissociation position.
- Refractive error has changed.

It is common for the cover test to be carried out pre-refraction with the patient wearing their glasses if they use them and subjective measures of heterophoria are performed post-refraction with the patient wearing a trial frame and correcting trial lenses. However, those practitioners that use a phoropter may prefer to use subjective measurements of heterophoria pre-refraction with the patient's current prescription dialled in and also post-refraction with the new prescription in place.

The MW does not give any information on the presence of a heterotropia and should only be used on patients with some level of binocularity.

The MW is designed to work at 30cm. The patient looks through two eye slit holes and the presence of the septa means that separate views seen by RE and LE i.e. different targets are presented to each eye so fusion cannot occur. The RE sees arrows while the LE sees tangent scales. The MW is used for quantifying near phoria.

Procedure
Explain: This test checks how well your eye muscles work together when looking at near objects.
Ask patient to wear appropriate correction with correct near papillary distance.
Room lights should be on with a local light source directed towards the MW targets (arrows, numbers) if required.
Ask: Please look through these horizontal eye slits. Can you see the red and white arrows and numbers?

As before, encourage patient to see both targets and stop test if one eye is suppressing

To measure horizontal phoria ask: Which white number does the white arrow point to? See Figure 17.

To measure vertical phoria ask: Which red number does the red arrow point to? See Figure 18.

To measure cyclophoria ask: Is the red bar horizontal? See Figure 19.

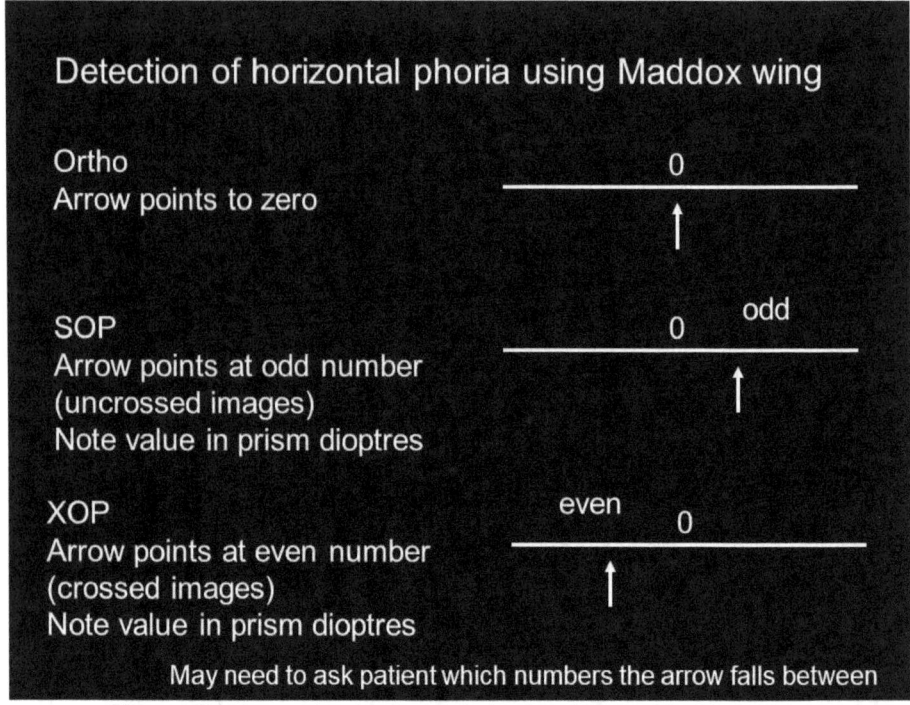

Figure 17 Measuring horizontal phoria with the Maddox wing.

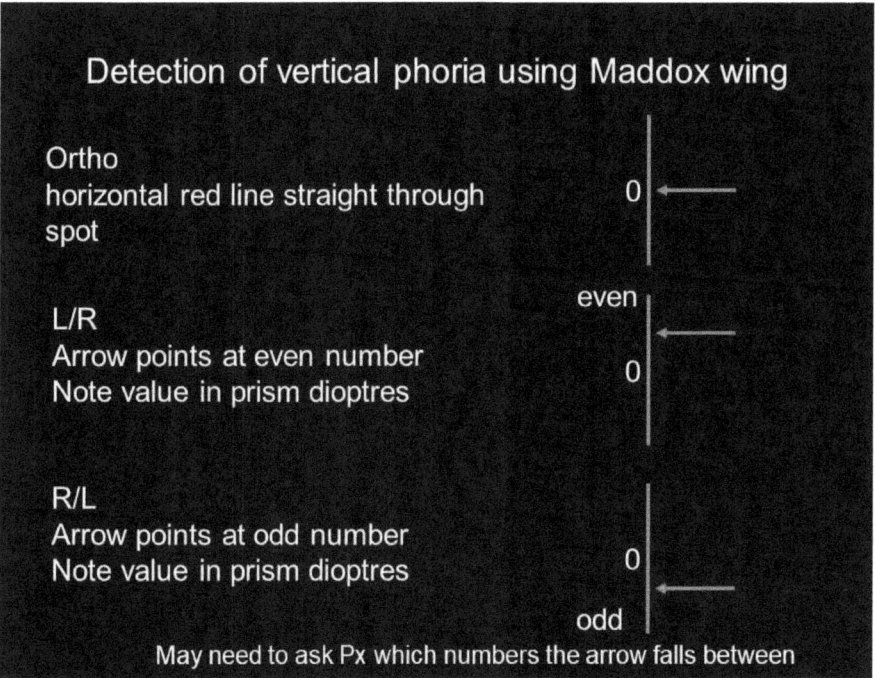

Figure 18 Measuring vertical phoria with the Maddox wing.

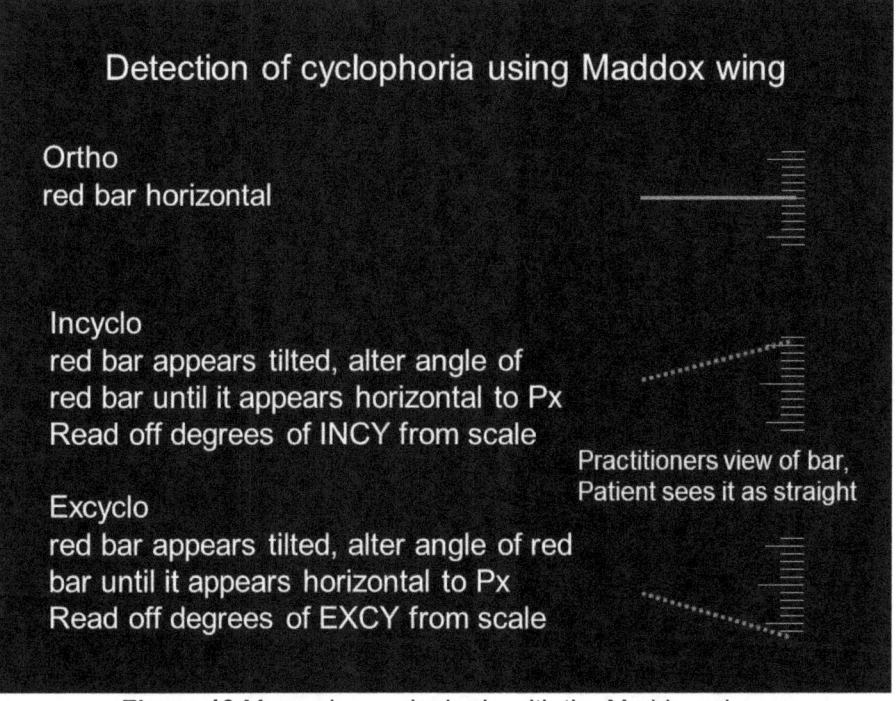

Figure 19 Measuring cyclophoria with the Maddox wing.

Hints and tips
Numbers and arrows are poor stimulus for accommodation and therefore:
Exophoria is overestimated and esophoria is underestimated.
Still useful for vertical and cyclophoria.
Arguably useful for patients over 55 years of age.
Septa are seen by each eye so dissociation is not full.
Tangent scales only designed for standard PD.

Most common errors:
> Allowing patient to adopt CHP.
> Assessing phoria in patient without binocular vision.
> Incorrect PD in trial frame.

Recording findings

MW – record the test carried out

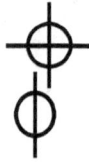
 – horizontal and vertical orthophoria

1 R/L – horizontal orthophoria, 1$^\Delta$ R hyperphoria

3 SOP-3Δ esophoria with vertical orthophoria

3 SOP 1 R/L   3$^\Delta$ esophoria with 1$^\Delta$ R hyperphoria

RE suppression – test not carried out

Chapter 25 Distance and near Mallett Unit

Introduction
Ideally, binocular single vision occurs when both visual axes are aligned with the object so that an image falls on each fovea. However, binocular single vision is still possible if visual axis misalignment is small enough to fall within Panum's fusional area. This misalignment is referred to as fixation disparity (FD) or retinal slip (slip). The amount of prism required to remove FD has traditionally been called the associated phoria, strictly meaning that there should be no dissociation (disruption of fusion) at all so that the eyes are measured in their active position. In practice, some degree of dissociation is essential and the term aligning sphere or aligning prism has been advocated. There are two main types of Mallett Unit: one used in the assessment of vision problems associated with near vision tasks of which there are various versions. The other used mainly at 6 m when visual discomfort is experienced when carrying out distance vision tasks. Both Mallett Units allow the detection of fixation disparity while the only the near unit can be used to detect foveal suppression associated with heterophoria and anomalous retinal correspondence (ARC) associated with small angle comitant strabismus. There is a distance foveal suppression test but in our experience this is rarely found in general optometric practice.

Use
People sometimes present to optometrists complaining of headache, eye ache, tired and sore eyes, poor concentration, poor performance at school and visual discomfort especially when reading, writing or carrying out VDU work. Symptoms are often associated with near tasks but sometimes occur at distance, and in particular when driving or with board work. With this clinical scenario many optometrists would test for the presence of fixation disparity, and if present, use small spherical lenses or prisms to neutralise the disparity in an attempt to reduce or totally alleviate symptoms. Where appropriate, small prisms or spheres can be incorporated into the prescription and worn as conventional spectacles to significantly improve visual comfort and relieve asthenopia.

Design
The Nonius (line) targets are the only part of target seen monocularly and these become displaced with FD because they adopt oculocentric visual direction. The lines are back illuminated so are not easily suppressed. Red lines for distance (accommodative lead) green for near (accommodative lag).

The central targets (letters OXO) and the peripheral surround are seen binocularly and so adopt an egocentric visual direction; this ensures minimal dissociation so that the binocular status is measured under more natural viewing conditions than the cover test, MR and MW. Binocular vision is completely undisturbed allowing subsequent tests to be undertaken under optimal conditions.

Procedure
Distance Mallett unit
Room lights on.
Explain 'This test helps determine whether your eye muscles are causing eye strain when you are looking in the distance'.
Turn Mallett on with OXO horizontal. See Figure 20.
Use appropriate distance refractive correction with correct PD.
Demonstrate alignment of strips without polarising visor in place by asking: Please look at the X in the middle of the OXO. Do you see two red strips, one above and one below the X? Are the strips exactly in line with each other and are both pointing to the middle of the X?
Attach the polarising visor to the front of the trial frame.
Occlude the RE and ask: Can you see the upper strip now?
Adjust the visor so that the LE sees the upper strip.
Remove the occluder form the RE and ask: Can you still see two red strips?
If deep suppression present, stop test and record findings.
Ask: Are the strips in line with the centre of the X?
If misaligned, align strip(s) with weakest sphere or prism.
Repeat with OXO vertical and strips horizontal.
Check for cyclodeviation by asking: Do the strips appear tilted?

Near Mallett unit
Room lights on, position local lighting to illuminate the front of the Mallett unit.
Explain: This test helps determine whether your eye muscles are causing eye strain when you are reading.
Turn Mallett on with OXO horizontal. See Figure 21.
Appropriate near refractive correction worn with correct PD.
Demonstrate alignment of strips without polarizing visor in place by asking: Please look at the X in the middle of the OXO. Do you see two green strips, one above and one below the OXO? Are the strips exactly in line with each other and pointing to the middle of the X?
Attach the polarising visor to the front of the trial frame.
Point at text that matches patient's near VA, ask: Please read this paragraph.
Occlude RE and ask: Can you see the upper strip now?
Adjust polarizing visor so that the LE sees the upper strip.
Remove the occluder and ask: Can you still see green strips?
If deep suppression present, stop test and record findings.
Ask: Are the strips in line with the middle of the X?
If misaligned, align strip(s) with weakest prism or sphere.
Repeat with OXO vertical and strips horizontal.
Check for cyclodeviation by asking: Do the strips appear tilted?

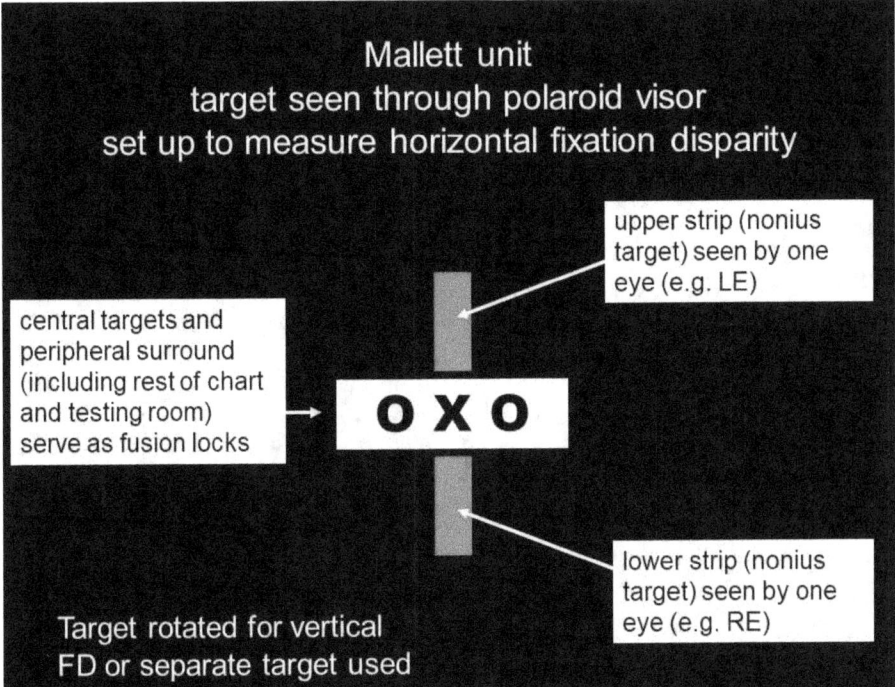

Figure 20 Detecting horizontal fixation disparity with the distance Mallett Unit.

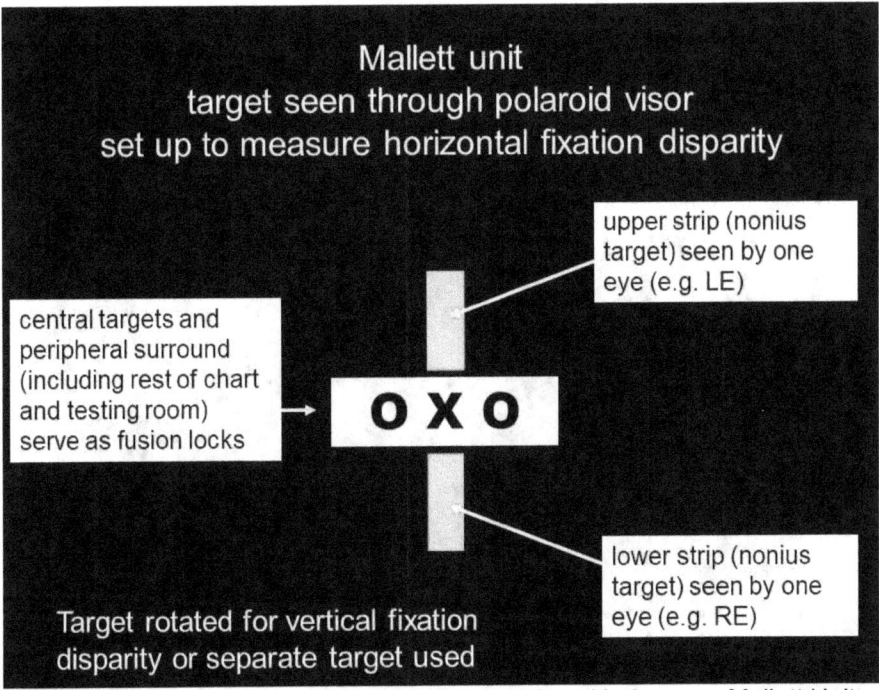

Figure 21 Detecting horizontal fixation disparity with the near Mallett Unit.

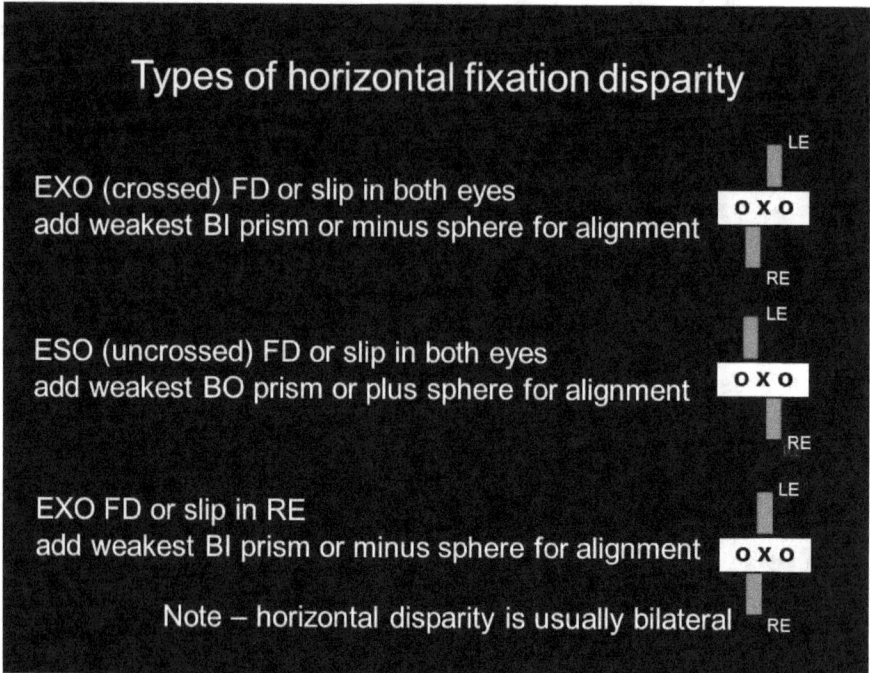

Figure 22 Types of horizontal fixation disparity (same for the near Mallett Unit). EXO exophoria, ESO esophoria, FD fixation disparity, BI base-in, BO base out

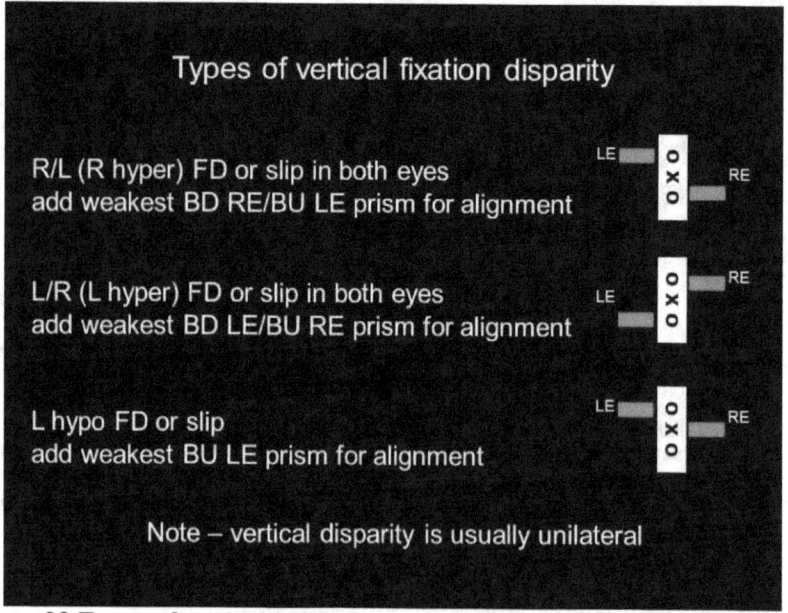

Figure 23 Types of vertical fixation disparity (same for the near Mallett Unit). hyper hyperphoria, hypo hypophoria, FD fixation disparity, BD base-down, BU base-up

Art of Clinical Practice in Optometry

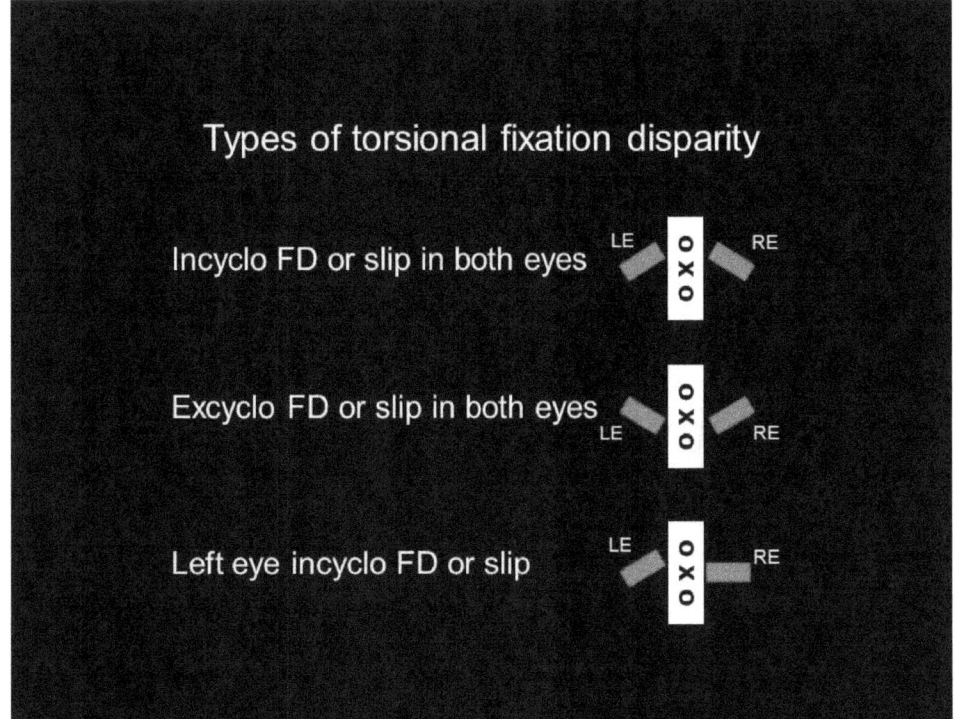

Figure 24 Types of torsional fixation disparity (same for the near Mallett Unit). Incyclo incyclophoria, Excyclo excyclophoria, FD fixation disparity

See Figures 22, 23 and 24 for types of fixation disparity. The types are the same for distance and near.

Recording findings
Mallett – record the test carried out.
No FD – no fixation disparity.
1 ESO RE – 1Δ ESO slip found in RE only.
½ EXO – ½Δ EXO slip found in both eyes.
2 EXO ½ R/L – 2Δ EXO slip with 1Δ R hyper slip both eyes.
RE suppression – test not carried out.
Also record the type of refractive correction worn during the test.

Expected findings
No slip and no rotation.

Hints and tips
The general lighting must be above average as some light is lost through the polarising visor.
A small prism or sphere should always be tried first, in spite of the presence of a large heterophoria.

When using the near Mallett Unit after changes in prism or spheres patients should be asked to read a few lines of the near text, to stabilise accommodation and convergence.

Exoslip
Adult patient: may respond best to base-in prism.
Young patient: minus sphere may work or consider orthoptic training to improve prism fusional reserves.

Esoslip
Base-out prism often best solution.
Plus sphere for near slip (do not over plus!!).
Consider orthoptic training to improve fusional reserves in children.
Vertical/torsional slip
Correct horizontal slip first, then vertical, torsional may resolve.
If prescribing prism add to one eye if unilateral slip; split between both eyes if bilateral slip.

Chapter 26 Direct ophthalmoscopy-anterior segment examination

Introduction
Direct ophthalmoscopy is the most commonly used ocular examination technique in general optometric practice. To undertake successful ophthalmoscopy it is essential that both the practitioner and the patient are comfortable. The patient will be more co-operative when relaxed and the practitioner will be more successful if the chair is adjusted to avoid stooping.

Use
This technique is used to assess the health of the eye, to identify abnormalities or the need for further investigation.

Procedure
Instruct the patient to look at a distant target, the white spot light on the vision chart is best and advise them to keep still and concentrate on this spot and to 'pretend' they can still see it even if you obscure it with your head.
The patient also needs to be given permission to blink and breathe as required.
It is best if the examination is conducted in subdued lighting to improve contrast of the ocular structures.
Your left eye and left hand should be used to examine the patient's left eye.
The field of view of the fundus is increased the closer you are to the patient's eye; so for low myopes and low hyperopes it is best to remove their glasses.
For myopes and hyperopes above ± 3.00DS and for astigmatism above 2.50DC it is advisable to keep the glasses on in order to overcome problems associated with magnification, minification and distortion, respectively.
Using a large diameter aperture and looking around the side of the ophthalmoscope examine the external features of the eye; this includes lashes, lid margins, palpebral conjunctiva, sclera, the colour of the iris and the size and regularity of the pupil.
Dial in a +10DS lens and examine the eye from 10cm.
Study the red reflex in particular as this provides an excellent way to detect any opacity of the media; dark patches or irregularity of the normal uniform red reflex denotes opacity of the cornea, anterior chamber or the vitreous.
Look out for a Mittendorf dot, which is a small congenital opacity on the posterior surface of the crystalline lens often present in normal healthy eyes.
The position of an opacity can be inferred from its parallax with respect to the pupil. Whilst examining the red-reflex, ask the patient to look up or down slightly.
If, when the patient looks up the opacity appears to move in the same direction within the red-reflex then it must lie anterior to the pupil plane (i.e. the cornea or the anterior chamber).

One that remains stationary must be in the plane of the pupil, and one that moves in the opposite direction to that of the patient's gaze must lie posterior to the pupil plane (that is, the posterior lens or vitreous).

The same effect can be achieved if the practitioner moves slightly from side to side with the patient remaining still.

Hints and tips
During ophthalmoscopy it is advisable to keep both your eyes open and suppress the image from the non-viewing eye; it may take some practice to accomplish this.

Recording findings
For R and LE:
Lashes – external hordeolum.
Lid/lid margin – debris.
Conjunctiva – pink/red.
Sclera – blue patch.
Iris – pigment loss.
Cornea – arcus senilis.
Anterior chamber – hypopyon.
Lens – cataract.

Expected findings
For R and LE:
Lashes – clean.
Lid/lid margin – healthy.
Conjunctiva – healthy.
Sclera – healthy.
Iris – colour.
Cornea – clear.
Anterior chamber – optically empty.
Lens – clear.

Chapter 27 Direct ophthalmoscopy-posterior segment examination

Introduction
Direct ophthalmoscopy is commonly used to assess the health of the eye.

Use
When evaluating the posterior pole the direct ophthalmoscope is used to assess the vitreous and retina, and to identify abnormalities or the need for further investigation. Abnormalities picked up in the posterior segment can be more thoroughly examined through dilated pupils using slit lamp or head mounted indirect ophthalmoscopy.

Procedure
Posterior segment examination usually follows on from assessment of the anterior segment.
Slowly move closer to the patient and at the same time gradually reduce the power of the lens in the wheel and focus on the crystalline lens, the vitreous and finally the fundus.
The power of lens necessary to focus on the fundus will depend on any patient and observer uncompensated refractive error and patient or observer accommodation.
Once a blood vessel on the fundus has been located then move along it and locate the point at which it branches and move your field of view in the direction in which the apex of the branch is pointing.
By moving along a blood vessel in this manner the optic disc will be located.
Consider the colour, clarity of margins and the cup if there is one.
Differentiate between a colour cup and a contour cup.
Note the presence of any pigment, choroidal or scleral crescents around the disc.
Retinal blood vessels should be examined in each quadrant after locating the disc; the veins are relatively large and dark red, whilst the arteries are relatively thin and pale.
Return to the disc and move nasally to view along the patient's visual axis.
In this position the fixation target will be obscured, the pupil will constrict and there will be some troublesome corneal reflections.
These factors make the macula a difficult area to visualise and it may be useful to use a smaller aperture beam.
The macula is the area between the superior and inferior temporal blood vessel arcades centred on the fovea.
Finally, ask the patient to look in the eight cardinal directions to allow a view of the peripheral fundus- 'look up' to see the superior periphery and so on.
In a young patient with a large pupil the equator of the eye will be accessible.

Adjust the lens in the wheel slightly as the periphery is closer to the observer than the optic disc requiring more focusing power (plus lens).

Hints and tips
Choose and appropriate fixation target for the subject.
Make sure the working distance is around 1 to 1.5 cm.
Use the appropriate aperture size or the various internal structures.
Position the ophthalmoscope to avoid making contact with the patient's face.
The practitioner should avoid embarrassing the patient with an inappropriate body posture.
The view of the peripheral retina is greatly advanced when the patient is asked to look in different positions of gaze.

Recording findings
Vitreous – floaters.
Neural retinal rim – pale nasal quadrant.
Disc margins – poorly defined.
Cup to disc ratio – value of ratio.
Crescents – choroidal.
Disc anomalies/abnormalities – tilting.
Vessels – tortuosity.
Fundus – pigmented.
Macula – haemorrhage.

Expected findings
Vitreous – clear.
Neural retinal rim – pink.
Disc margins – well defined.
Cup to disc ratio – (value of ratio).
Crescents – none, choroidal, scleral.
Disc anomalies/abnormalities – none.
Vessels – ¾ artery to vein ratio.
Fundus – healthy.
Macula – foveal reflex present.

Chapter 28 External and anterior eye examination using direct illumination

Introduction
Slit lamp examination of the lids, lashes, conjunctiva, sclera and cornea is important during contact lens fitting and aftercare and for those patients when symptoms or signs suggest the problem may lie with these ocular structures.

Diffuse illumination
This refers to a wide beam that is directed obliquely for general scanning with low magnification in order to maximise the field of view. It is not necessary to have a neutral density filter in place although this may be useful if the patient is photosensitive.

Slit lamp set up
- Coupled
- 30 to 60 degrees beam angle
- 3-4 mm beam width
- Maximum beam height
- No filter
- Medium illumination
- 10X magnification.

Procedure
Position the microscope directly in front of the eye, with the beam at an angle of 60 degrees, and the illumination system and focus on the temporal part of the eye.
Ask the patient to look along the side of the slit lamp.
When examining the patient's right eye the practitioners left ear could be used as a fixation target.
The red fixation light that is attached to most modern slit lamps can be used to move the eye under investigation into any required position.
Use the joystick to scan along the lower lid of the closed eye.
Scan across to the midline and then swing the beam across to the nasal part of the eye and scan back across to the midline.
The procedure should be repeated for the closed upper lid.
Lower and upper lid margins should also be examined with the eye open.
The lower bulbar and palpebral conjunctiva, sclera and cornea can be examined on the open eye by retracting and everting the lower lid with a forefinger.
The patient should be informed of contact prior to touching any part of the eye.
Conjunctiva, sclera and cornea between the lids and then the area beneath the upper lid can be examined in a similar manner.

The upper lid will have to be retracted in order to view the upper bulbar conjunctiva, sclera and cornea.

Hints and tips
Because the beam width is wide and the light is bright some patients may find this technique uncomfortable and it may be necessary to place a neutral density filter between the illumination and the patient.
This can be achieved in most slit lamps by 'dialling in the filter' within the illumination system or by manually flipping a filter over the bulb.
The intensity of the beam can be reduced without sacrificing clarity of view for the examiner.

Novice observers often:
- Do not realise that the beam is out of click stop and cannot focus the illumination directly on the eye.
- Use too high illumination with can be uncomfortable for the patient and result in 'washing out' features of interest with too much light.
- Use too high a magnification which results in loss of perspective of relative structures and a tendency to over interpret normal findings as abnormal.

It is important to shift the illumination arm from one side of the eye to the other when the corneal apex is reached in order to obtain an adequate view of all aspects of the anterior segment.

Recording findings
Diffuse illumination is used to observe the lids and lashes in order to detect the presence and to determine:
- Type of blepharitis
- Red/pink or crusty lid margins
- Meibomian gland dysfunction
- Internal and external hordeolum
- Lesions that may be neoplastic.
- Areas of interest can be further examined by increasing the magnification and narrowing the beam.

Bulbar and palpebral conjunctiva can be investigated with a narrower beam for conjunctival follicles and papillae, hyperaemia and injection, and any mucus or discharge.

This aids in the differential diagnosis of:
- Bacterial, viral, and allergic conjunctivitis
- Degenerative lesions of the conjunctiva such as pingeculae and pterygia can also be evaluated and monitored for change
- The sclera can be examined for redness, discoloration, thinning and trauma.
- Differential diagnosis between conjunctival and scleral inflammation can be made.
- The cornea can be assessed for gross abnormalities due to trauma, oedema or ulcer.

SECTION 4 FURTHER INVESTIGATION

Chapter 29 Pulsair™ non-contact tonometer calibration

Chapter 30 Pulsair™ non-contact tonometer procedure

Chapter 31 Goldmann tonometer calibration

Chapter 32 Perkins tonometer calibration

Chapter 33 Drug instillation

Chapter 34 Perkins and Goldmann tonometer procedure

Chapter 35 Visual field analysis patient set up

Chapter 36 Goldmann perimetry

Chapter 37 Humphrey visual field analyser

Chapter 38 Gross perimetry-confrontation and peripheral fields

Chapter 39 Henson Pro visual field analyser

Chapter 40 Ishihara colour vision test

Chapter 41 City University colour vision test

Chapter 42 Amsler grid

Chapter 43 Pelli-Robson Contrast Test

Chapter 44 Modified monocular indirect ophthalmoscopy

Chapter 45 Head mounted indirect ophthalmoscopy

Chapter 46 Slit lamp biomicroscopy

Chapter 47 Slit-lamp ophthalmoscopy with negative lenses

Chapter 48 Diagnostic contact lens and gonioscopy

Chapter 49 Examination of the anterior chamber

Chapter 50 Examination of the iris

Chapter 51 Examination of the vitreous

Chapter 29 Pulsair™ non-contact tonometer calibration

Introduction
This is a hand held instrument, which uses air pressure to applanate the cornea. Rather than measuring the pressure indirectly by recording the time taken to applanate, the Pulsair uses a transducer to directly measure the air pressure at the point at which the cornea is flattened.

Only when the tonometer is at the correct distance and properly aligned with respect to the patient's cornea, will the image of the corneal reflex fall onto three photodetectors in such a way that more light falls onto the two outer detectors than the central one. At the moment that the instrument senses that the contrast between the sum of the outer and the centre detectors is correct, a valve on the air reservoir automatically opens releasing air onto the patient's eye.

The increasing pulse of air decreases the corneal curvature until it is eventually flattened. At this moment more light falls on the central detector than the sum of the outer two. When this happens the pressure transducer, which is connected directly to the pneumatic system, samples the pulse pressure and the result is digitally displayed in mmHg. Consult the manual for your particular version of the Keeler Pulsair.

Procedure
Switch the instrument on and ensure it is correctly calibrated:
- Firing the demo button once will give a value of 30, firing it twice will give a value of 50 if the machine is calibrated
- Any other values means that the instrument is out of calibration and should not be used.

Chapter 30 Pulsair™ non-contact tonometer procedure

Introduction
This is a hand held instrument which uses air pressure to applanate the cornea. Rather than measuring the pressure indirectly by recording the time taken to applanate, the Pulsair uses a transducer to directly measure the air pressure at the point at which the cornea is flattened.

Only when the tonometer is at the correct distance and properly aligned with respect to the patient's cornea, will the image of the corneal reflex fall onto three photodetectors in such a way that more light falls onto the two outer detectors than the central one. At the moment that the instrument senses that the contrast between the sum of the outer and the centre detectors is correct, a valve on the air reservoir automatically opens releasing air onto the patient's eye.

The increasing pulse of air decreases the corneal curvature until it is eventually flattened. At this moment more light falls on the central detector than the sum of the outer two. When this happens the pressure transducer, which is connected directly to the pneumatic system, samples the pulse pressure and the result is digitally displayed in mmHg. Consult the manual for your particular version of the Keeler Pulsair.

Procedure
Explain to the patient what you are going to do.
Ask the patient to hold their hand up to the nozzle.
Press the demo button for demonstration.
Position the patient comfortably.
Press the set/reset button.
Place the nozzle about 2 cm away from the eye, holding the instrument steady.
Instruct the patient to look at the red dot.
Align the red reflex in the centre of the cornea by viewing directly.
Looking through the eyepiece, adjust the focus by moving in and out until you see the two red rectangles.
The instrument should automatically fire if you are aligned correctly.
If there is a delay of more than 30 seconds the light will go out and the set/reset button will have to be pressed again.
Repeat stages 5-10, three more times, record all four readings and then average.
Repeat for the other eye.
Record the type of instrument used and the time the measurements were taken.

Hints and tips
It may take some time to become proficient in aligning this instrument.

Recording findings
R 23, 24, 25, 25 Av. 24.5 mmHg.
L 25, 26, 25, 26 Av 25.5 mmHg.

Expected findings
R 14, 16, 16, 17 Av. 15.5 mmHg.
L 15, 17, 16, 16 Av 16.0 mmHg.

Chapter 31 Goldmann tonometer calibration

Introduction
The Goldmann applanation tonometer (GAT) consists of an applanating probe and weight loaded lever system, which is placed on a slit lamp mount. The applanating probe is a hollow conical shaped cylinder, containing a pair of prisms with their apices together. The end of the probe is brought into contact with the anaesthetised cornea is made. When contact is made, the observer views the applanated area (which is made visible by the instillation of fluorescein) directly through the probe with the microscope. The force is then adjusted until the applanated area has a diameter of 3.06 mm.

The prisms in the probe have the effect of shifting the upper half of the field of view to the left, and the lower half to the right, so that the centres of the two halves are separated by a distance of exactly 3.06 mm. The applanated area is therefore seen as two semicircles. When the applanated area is exactly 3.06 mm the inner edges of the semicircles will be in contact. Care must be taken to ensure that the dividing line between the two prisms bisects the applanated area.

The variable force required to flatten the cornea is applied by the means of a simple lever system employing an eccentrically placed weight. This avoids the problem of wear and tear variations that could be found in a spring tension system.

Use
Tonometry is the measurement of intraocular pressure (IOP) and the GAT is a device designed to measure IOP and assist in the detection and diagnosis and management of any ocular diseases that cause pressure to vary from the norm and in particular primary open angle glaucoma.

Calibration
To calibrate the Goldmann tonometer a metal rod is attached to the spring.
When the rod is in the null position equal amounts of rod are in front and behind the spring hence it creates no force on the spring.
When the spring load is now adjusted the probe will move forward when the reading is '0'. The rod is now pushed to the first mark backward.
This creates moments against the spring and tension has to be increased to 2 g before the probe moves forward.
A similar procedure is then carried out to the further mark, which will require 6g of spring tension before the probe moves forward.
The above describes the situation when calibration is perfect so that 1g of actual weight is represented by a reading of '1'.

Chapter 32 Perkins tonometer calibration

Introduction
This is a hand held version of the Goldmann tonometer. It uses a spring to exert a variable force upon the eye. It can be used with patients supine or erect. Since it lacks the control and security of a slit lamp, care must be taken to stabilise the instrument to ensure centration without causing damage. See Figure 25.

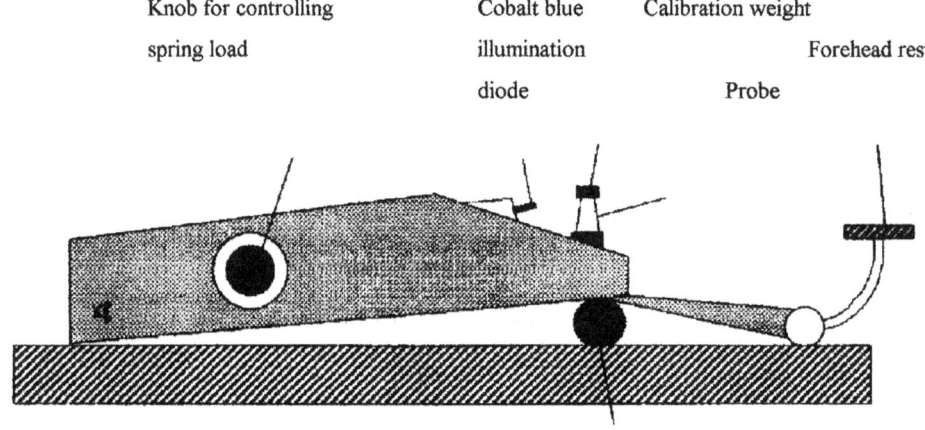

Figure 25 Perkins contact tonometer.

Use
The Perkins tonometer is used to measure IOP for the detection and management of glaucoma.

Calibration
To calibrate the Perkins tonometer it is placed so that the probe is vertical.
This is facilitated by use of a cylinder upon which the collar of the instrument rests.
The spring load is then altered until the probe rises, this should be at 0g of weight.
A calibration weight is then placed on top of the probe and the spring load increased until the probe and weight rise.
The probe should rise at 2 g and 5 g of weight when the lighter and heavier weights are placed on the probe respectively.
As with the Goldmann tonometer if the instrument reads lower or higher it may still be used provided the calibration error is the same at each weight.

Chapter 33 Drug instillation

Introduction
Some patients will require the instillation of eye drops as part of the eye examination. The administration of topical eye drops should be done in a safe, effective and appropriate manner.

Use
To dilate the pupil to enable enhanced fundoscopy.
To allow examination of the cornea and conjunctiva using fluorescein and blue light.
To allow cycloplegic refraction.
To allow contact tonometry

Procedure
Check it is the correct drug, correct strength, correct eye (if instillation is only required for one eye, correct dose, check the expiry date of the medication has not been exceeded.
This will safeguard against wrongful administration.
Explain the procedure to the patient and the purpose of administration to obtain informed consent and co-operation.
Seat the patient with their head well supported.
Wash hands.
Ask patient to look up and gently pull down the lower lid to form a 'sac' to ensure safe technique, patient comfort and to avoid damage to the cornea.
Squeeze one drop into sac at the outer temporal area of the lower eyelid, taking care not to contaminate the bottle.
Ask the patient to close their eye for 30 seconds. This will aid the absorption of the eye drops and minimise discomfort to the patient.
Instruct the patient how to occlude the punctum by gently pressing on the medial canthus for a minimum of one minute, immediately after the instillation of eye drops. This helps to minimise systemic absorption of eye drops, is essential in some cases and advisable in others especially in the case of children.
When practising punctal occlusion the patient should wash their hands before and after the instillation of any eye drops.
If more than one type of eye drop is required at the same time, a space of at least five minutes between the first and the second is recommended.
Repeat procedure to other eye if necessary, washing hands in between to comply with safe technique and to minimise the risk of contamination.
Dispose of any waste materials.

Recordings
Drug name, strength, eyes applied to, expiry date and batch number.

Chapter 34 Perkins and Goldmann tonometer procedure

Introduction
This is a hand held version of the Goldmann tonometer. It uses a spring to exert a variable force upon the eye. It can be used with patients supine or erect. Since it lacks the control and security of a slit lamp, care must be taken to stabilise the instrument to ensure centration without causing damage.

Use
The Perkins tonometer is used to measure IOP for the detection and in the management of glaucoma.

Procedure
Turn the instrument on and ensure that the light is bright and shining at the end of the probe (if not then change the batteries).
Position the patient correctly, with the head supported behind if possible.
Wash hands.
Place a disposable probe in the holder ensuring that the bi-prism is horizontal. If there is >3DC, then the applanated area will be oval rather than round, leading to possible misreading the scale. To record an accurate IOP the mires must be equal in shape and size. This can be achieved by rotating the prisms to bisect the short axis of the oval or the flattest meridian should be placed at 43 degrees to the axis of the cone. Check the drug, dosage and expiry date of a Minim® of 0.5% Proxymetacaine with fluorescein.
Explain to the patient the procedure.
Instil one drop into the lower fornix of each eye.
Even if the intra-ocular pressure of one eye is to be recorded, instilling anaesthetic into both eyes will help to suppress the blink reflex.
Position the patient, make any adjustments to your position and explain what you are going to do.
Turn the wheel that controls the force of the probe to 1.6 (16 mmHg).
Approach quickly to just beyond lash plane.
Align laterally and vertically, before going onto corneal cap.
Move quickly but smoothly to the cornea.
Small movements on cornea are acceptable but take care do not scrape entire area.
Too little pressure, no overlap of mires.
Just right mires touch on inner portion of rings, mires should pulsate at appropriate measurement.
Too much pressure, excessive overlap.

Record the IOP values along with the instrument type and time the measurements were made.

Hints and tips
Probe too high-move down towards larger semi-circle.
Probe too low-move up towards larger semi-circle.
If within 1/2 of circle of probe mires, slide over cornea 2-3 mm.
If outside circle, remove from eye, readjust and try again.
Mires too thick- gives reading too high and therefore wait a minute for some of the fluorescein to dissipate.
Mires too thin-gives reading too low and therefore add more fluorescein.

Recording findings
Perkins R 24, L 25 mmHg.

Expected findings
R and L 16 mmHg.

Goldmann applanation tonometry
Introduction
The Goldmann applanation tonometer (GAT) consists of an applanating probe and weight loaded lever system, which is placed on a slit lamp mount. The applanating probe is a hollow conical shaped cylinder, containing a pair of prisms with their apices together. The end of the probe is brought into contact with the anaesthetised cornea. When contact is made, the observer views the applanated area (made visible by instillation of fluorescein) directly through the probe with the microscope. The force is adjusted until the applanated area has a diameter of 3.06 mm.

The prisms in the probe have the effect of shifting the upper half of the field of view to the left, and the lower half to the right, so that the centres of the two halves are separated by a distance of exactly 3.06 mm. The applanated area is therefore seen as two semicircles. When the applanated area is exactly 3.06 mm the inner edges of the semicircles will be in contact. Care must be taken to ensure that the dividing line between the two prisms bisects the applanated area.

The variable force required to flatten the cornea is applied by the means of a simple lever system employing an eccentrically placed weight. This avoids the problem of wear and tear variations that could be found in a spring tension system.

Use
Tonometry is the measurement of intra-ocular pressure (IOP) and the GAT is a device designed to measure IOP and assist in the detection and diagnosis and management of any ocular diseases that cause pressure to vary from the norm and in particular primary open angle glaucoma.

Procedure
Place a disposable probe in the holder ensuring that the bi-prism is horizontal. If there is >3DC, then the applanated area will be oval rather than round, leading to

possible misreading the scale. To record an accurate IOP the mires must be equal in shape and size. This can be achieved by rotating the prisms to bisect the short axis of the oval or the flattest meridian should be placed at 43 degrees to the axis of the cone.

Attach the Goldmann tonometer to the slit lamp.
Position the patient correctly on the slit-lamp, ensuring they are at the correct height and comfortable.
Wash hands.
Check the drug, dosage and expiry date of a Minim® of 0.5% Proxymetacaine with fluorescein.
Explain to the patient what is going to happen.
Instil one drop into the lower fornix of each eye.
Even if the IOP from only one eye is to be taken, instilling anaesthetic into both eyes will help reduce the blink reflex.
Position the patient at the slit lamp again and explain the procedure.
Set up the illumination system so that it is positioned temporally with maximum intensity blue light (cobalt blue filter must be used in order to see the fluorescein) shining on the tonometer tip.
Turn the wheel that controls the force of the probe to 1 (16 mmHg).
Approach quickly to just beyond lash plane. Align laterally and vertically to be in line with the centre of the cornea.
Look from the temporal side and move quickly but smoothly forward to make contact with the centre of the cornea.
Alternatively look through the microscope gently move the probe forward until two green semi-circles are observed indicating that contact has been made with the cornea.
Small movements of the probe on the cornea are acceptable and area almost always necessary to achieve alignment with the corneal centre.
When the probe is correctly aligned with the corneal centre, adjust the dial until semicircles are touching and then take the reading from the adjustment dial.

Hints and tips
If one semi-circle is larger than the other move the probe while still in contact with the cornea away from the direction of the larger semi-circle, for example if the upper semi-circle is larger than the lower semi-circle then move the probe downwards slightly.
If a complete circle is seen then the tonometer tip is not near the centre of the cornea and it should be pulled back and the procedure started from the beginning.
Mires too thick-blot fluorescein, gives reading that is too high. Mires too thin-add fluorescein, gives reading that is too low.

Recording findings
Goldmann R 19, L 20 mmHg.

Expected findings
R and L 16 mmHg

Chapter 35 Visual field analysis patient set up

Introduction
One of the most important, but often forgotten parts of the visual field analysis is the setting up stage. Inadequate set up of the patient or the instrument or both is the most common cause for artefactual visual field defects.

Room Illumination
To gain repeatable and meaningful visual field results it is extremely important that the room illumination is always kept the same. The ideal is a completely blacked out room. In optometric practice this is not always possible, and visual field analyzers are often positioned in rooms were ambient illumination may fluctuate because of doors opening and inappropriate general lighting. If this is the case a slightly brighter room illumination and background luminance are best, so that the test is less sensitive to small fluctuations in ambient illumination. The most important factor is that the illumination used is always the same and is in accordance with the recommendations for the instrument being used. Room illumination should therefore be considered at the beginning of each session.

Background luminance
Each visual field instrument is designed to be used at a specified background luminance. Many of the more modem visual field instruments will adjust the background luminance to take account of room illumination; some have built in light meters that allow the background luminance to be adjusted. It is important that the recommended luminance for the instrument is known and that it is calibrated it at the beginning of each session if this is not done automatically.

Patient adaptation time
It can take up to half-an-hour for the eyes to adapt completely to darkness when a person enters a dim room from a very bright environment. Most adaptation, however, occurs in the first five minutes. It is important therefore to set the room and background luminance to the levels you are using for the test before you set up the patient so that they have time to adapt.

Seating the patient comfortably
The patient should be seated as comfortably as possible, squarely facing the screen, usually with their chin on a rest and forehead against a bar. Some instruments have a monitor that allows you to line up the eye; others have a mark for the level with the outer canthus. Each person is unique in size, and the chair, instrument and chin rest will all need to be adjusted to obtain the correct position. It is extremely important that the patient is seated comfortably.

Explain the test to the patient
Take your time to explain what is going to happen to the patient. This should include where they should look, what their responses should be and approximately how long the test will take. For example: This is a test to see what you are seeing out of the sides of your eyes. Throughout the test it is important that you look at the central spot(s) all the time. Always look at the spot straight ahead. Sometimes you will go for a period without seeing any lights in your side vision, this is all part of the test. If you need a rest at any time just let me know.

For multiple stimulus supra-threshold: Lights will flash around the side. There will be between 0 and 4 lights. When you see some lights flash I want you to tell me how many you thought you saw. Sometimes I will ask you where the lights flashed. If this happens describe where you thought you saw them in relation to a clock face.

For kinetic perimetry: Lights of different size and brightness will move in front of you from the outside. If you think you see a light coming press the button.

Determining what trial lens to use
Most visual field tests are set at 33cm from the patient's eyes. It is a near visual task and the patient must be corrected for that distance using full aperture trial lenses. It is not good practice to use the reading prescription because this may be set for a longer working distance. If bifocals are used then some of the stimulus presentations may be blurred when the patient looks through the distance portion. Measure the patient's distance correction. If they have a cylindrical power <1.00DC calculate the best vision sphere of the distance correction and add a near addition according to their age to obtain the best trial lens for visual field testing:

Age	Addition
<35 years	no addition
40-44 years	+1.50DS
45-49 years	+2.00DS
50-54 years	+2.50DS
55-59 years	+3.00DS
60-64 years	+3.50DS
>64 years	+4.00DS

For example, a 56 year old patient, distance spectacle prescription +1.00/-0.50 x 90 Best Vision Sphere = +0.75 plus +3.00DS for near, therefore use +3.75DS for the trial lens or if the cylinder is ≥ 1.00 use the exact distance spectacle prescription (including a cyl) plus the near add as above.

Occlude one eye
If previous tests indicate one eye has a better visual field or if VA testing indicates a better eye then test the better eye first.
Put the trial lens in the holder and line it and the patient up.
Bring the trial lens as close to the patient's eye as possible without touching the lashes. If a cylinder is used, the axis is recorded from a perspective of looking at the patient.

Chapter 36 Goldmann perimetry

Introduction
This technique is an example of kinetic perimetry during which a stimulus of known size and intensity is brought from a position outside the island of vision (where it cannot be seen) towards its centre until it is seen i.e. when it touches the island of vision. See Figure 26. This point represents the limit of the field for that stimulus. This is then repeated in different meridians.

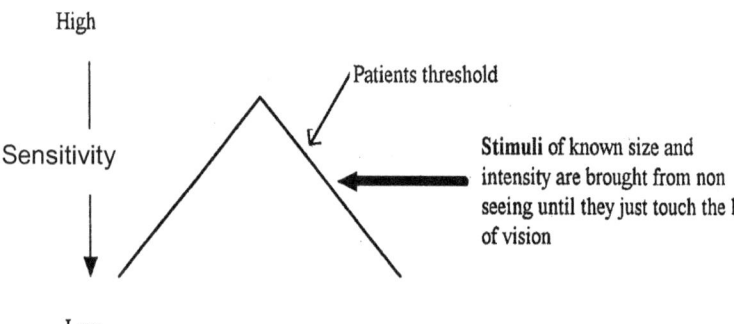

Figure 26 Kinetic perimetry and the hill of vision.

The Goldmann perimeter has the following characteristics:
- Extent of visual field tested - 180 degrees
- Test distance and type - 30 cm, bowl.
- Background luminance - 10 cd/m^2 calibrated manually using a light meter

Stimuli - the standard Goldmann instrument has six different sizes of stimuli, which are represented by Roman numerals:

Target	Size (area mm^2)
0	0.0625
I	0.25
II	1
III	4
IV	16
V	64

The instrument has four stimulus intensities that are obtained by placing neutral density filters in 0.5 log unit steps. These are represented by the numbers 1 to 4, with 4 being the brightest at 1000Asb. Intensities 3, 2 and 1 are obtained by placing 0.5, 1.0 and 1.5 log unit filters in front of the illuminating beam.

To give finer adjustment a second set of filters, 'a' to 'e', is incorporated in some systems. These correspond to 0.4, 0.3, 0.2, 0.1 and 0.0 log units. With a combination of the two sets of filters it is possible to change the intensity of the stimulus in 0.1 log steps. In practice however the second set of filters are rarely used, being set on 'e' (0.0 log units ND).

Filter	Log Units	Intensity (cd/m^2) Attenuation	Asb
4e	0.0	318	1000
3e	0.5	102	320
2e	1.0	31.8	100
1e	1.5	10.2	10.2

Fixation is monitored by direct observation through a telescope.

The Goldmann perimeter is a manual perimeter that allows examination of the field up to 90 degrees eccentricity around fixation. It uses a pantographic arm to connect the projector that produces the stimuli to the recording chart. The position of the pen held by the practitioner on the chart therefore corresponds to the position of the stimulus in the patient's visual field. The system is extremely flexible, allowing the perimetrist to move the stimuli in any direction at any speed in any position of the visual field. The stimuli being used are usually continuously on, although there is also a facility that allows the light to be presented briefly. This allows static checking of the central visual field. The results are recorded onto pre-printed chart paper. Different isopters are usually recorded using different coloured pencils. There is no means to electronically store results and analysis is by visual inspection.

Procedure
Reduce the room illumination.
Switch the instrument on; it should be calibrated at the beginning of each session.
Select appropriate refractive correction but do not put it in the lens holder yet.
Set up the patient with the selected first eye central and move the chin rest, chair and instrument so that the selected eye appears central in the telescopic viewing system.
Occlude the eye not being examined.
Explain the test to the patient and ensure they have the response button in their hand.
Choose a large bright stimulus to begin with e.g. V4e; this is done by sliding the three selection bars on the upper right hand side to the desired settings.
At the right hand side of the bowl there is a wheel and when this is pushed down the stimulus comes on.
Push the wheel down and show the patient the stimulus.

With the wheel still pushed down move the pen/stylus that is connected to the pantographic arm from the edge of the chart (non-seeing) steadily towards the centre of the chart until the patient notices the target.

Repeat this a few times to ensure reliability of responses so that you are sure the patient understands the test.

When the responses are repeatable mark the position of the stimulus when it is first seen by the patient with a pen on the chart.

Using this same V4e stimulus test along other meridians by moving around the chart testing every 15 degrees or so.

Each time mark the position at which the patient notices the target. It is important not to move in a circle all the time.

Test two or three consecutive meridians then jump to somewhere else on the chart.

Always test at either side of horizontal and vertical midlines, not along them

Repeat three or four meridians to gauge reliability of results and monitor fixation periodically

When 360 degrees have been tested join the dots on the chart together using a coloured pen to plot the V4e isopters.

Change the size of the stimulus to plot the next isopter. I4e is a smaller stimulus than V4e but has the same intensity.

Repeat the steps above using the I4e stimulus.

Use a different coloured pen to mark the chart.

Now change the intensity if the stimulus.

I2e is the same size as I4e but dimmer.

Repeat the above steps using the I2e stimulus to plot an isopter.

Use another coloured pen to mark the chart.

This isopter may cross into the central 30 degrees and trial lens should be placed in front of the patient's eye for anything that is plotted inside the central 30 degrees.

Repeat for the other eye.

Hints and tips
It is more important to test along 16 meridians well than 40 badly and tire the patient.

Recording findings
See Figures 27 and 28 for Goldmann plots depicting central visual field loss corresponding to the physiological defect associated with the optic nerve head (blind spot) and bilateral pathological peripheral field defects.

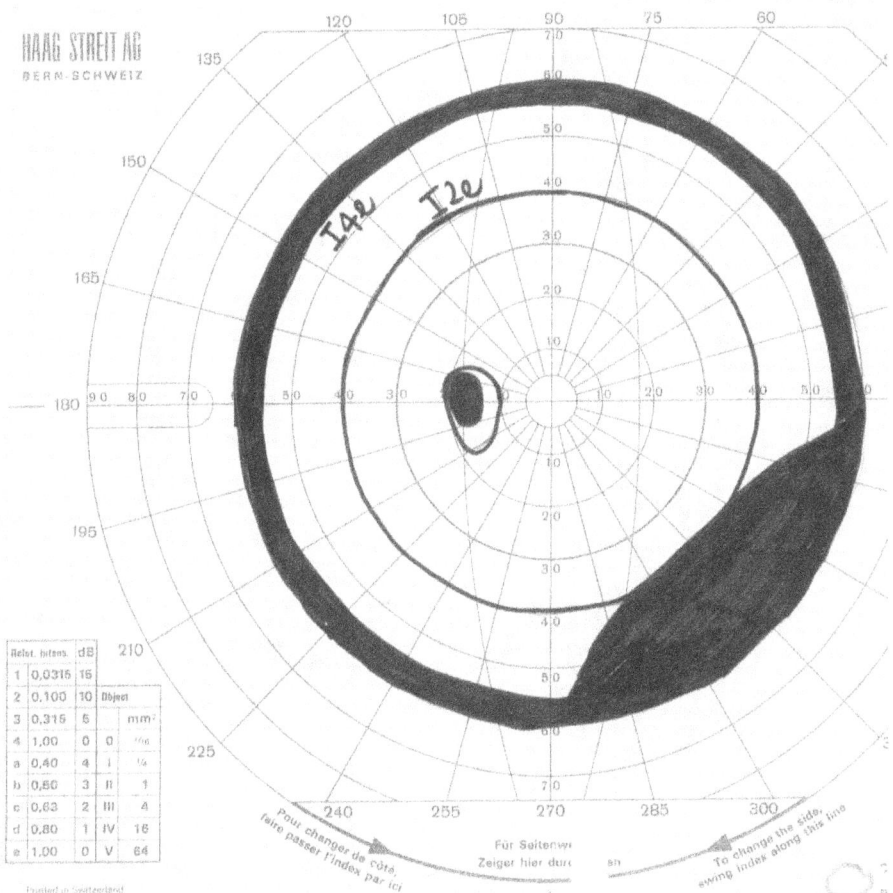

Figure 27 Blind spot and pathological peripheral field defect left eye.

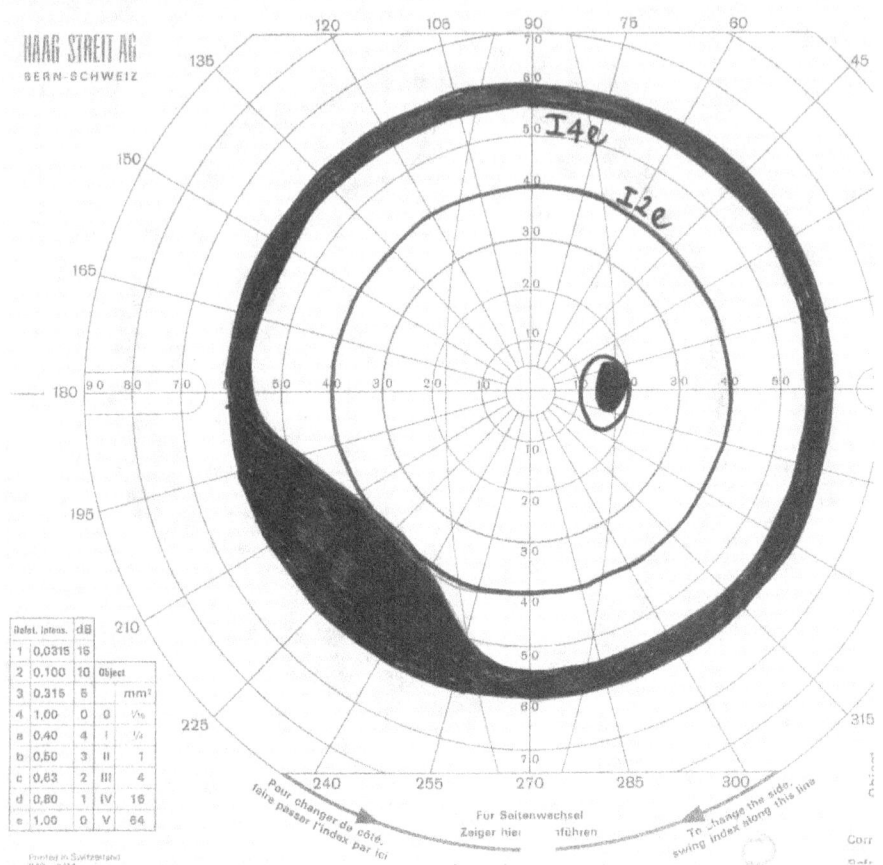

Figure 28 Blind spot and pathological peripheral field defects right eye.

Chapter 37 Humphrey visual field analyser

Introduction
The Humphrey visual field analyser is a bowl perimeter and stimuli are projected onto the bowl. In the full threshold examination strategy the threshold is estimated at a series of points. See Figure 29.

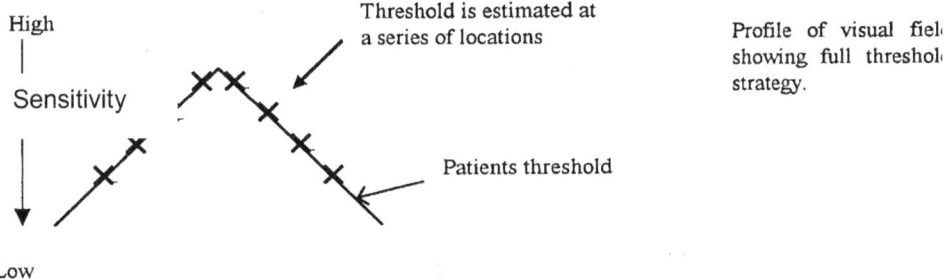

Figure 29 Threshold estimation for the Humphrey visual field analyser.

The Humphrey Visual Field Analyser offers many strategies. These vary depending on the model but can include single-stimulus threshold related and supra-threshold strategies. Some are quantified and some are designed specifically for glaucoma. It can include:

> Estermann test (used to assess driving fields)
> Peripheral visual field
> Tests designed to assess neurological defects
> Some models have kinetic strategies.

There are also many different full threshold strategies that vary according to the number and location of stimuli and whether they take into account results from previous examinations. A commonly used strategy is the 24-2 SITA program. Fixation is monitored using a video camera that relays images to the operators monitor. Fixation is also monitored periodically by presenting a stimulus in the region of the patient's blind spot. If fixation is accurate the stimulus will not be seen – this is called the Heijl-Krakau technique.

To assess the reliability of the patient's responses false positive and false negative responses are periodically tested for. On occasions the instrument makes a noise that is suggestive of stimuli presentation, but no stimuli are presented. If the patient presses the button indicating that they saw a stimulus then this is recorded as a *false positive* response. After the threshold of a few points has been assessed it goes back to those points and presents stimuli that are known to be above threshold. If the patient fails to respond then this is recorded as *a false negative* response. Results can be printed out in a variety of forms including grey scale and numeric formats. Data is also saved in the inbuilt computer for storage or recall for future analysis.

Use
The Humphrey visual field analyser can be used to screen for visual field defects in a normal population or patients who are at risk of primary open angle glaucoma or for patients who have suspected neurological lesions such as in multiple sclerosis. The system can also be used to monitor progression or reversal of visual field loss during treatment.

Procedure
Reduce the room illumination.
Switch the instrument on and allow it to self-calibrate.
Select appropriate correction (if required) and place it in the lens holder.
Enter patient details.
Select the required programme.
Set up the patient on the chin rest, with the selected first eye central and move the rest, chair and instrument so that the selected eye appears central on the display cross at the centre of the pupil with the eye located in the centre of the lens in use.
Occlude the eye not being examined.
Explain the test to the patient.
Start the test when everything is set up and ready and the patient has the response button.
Repeat for the other eye.
When the test is complete save and print the results.

Hints and tips
In order to avoid artefactual field defects make sure that the patient and instrument are set up appropriately.
Encourage the patient as the test proceeds.

Recording findings
See Figure 30 for a Humphrey plot depicting a normal visual field for the RE and Figure 31 for a Humphrey plot depicting an inferior visual field defect in the LE.

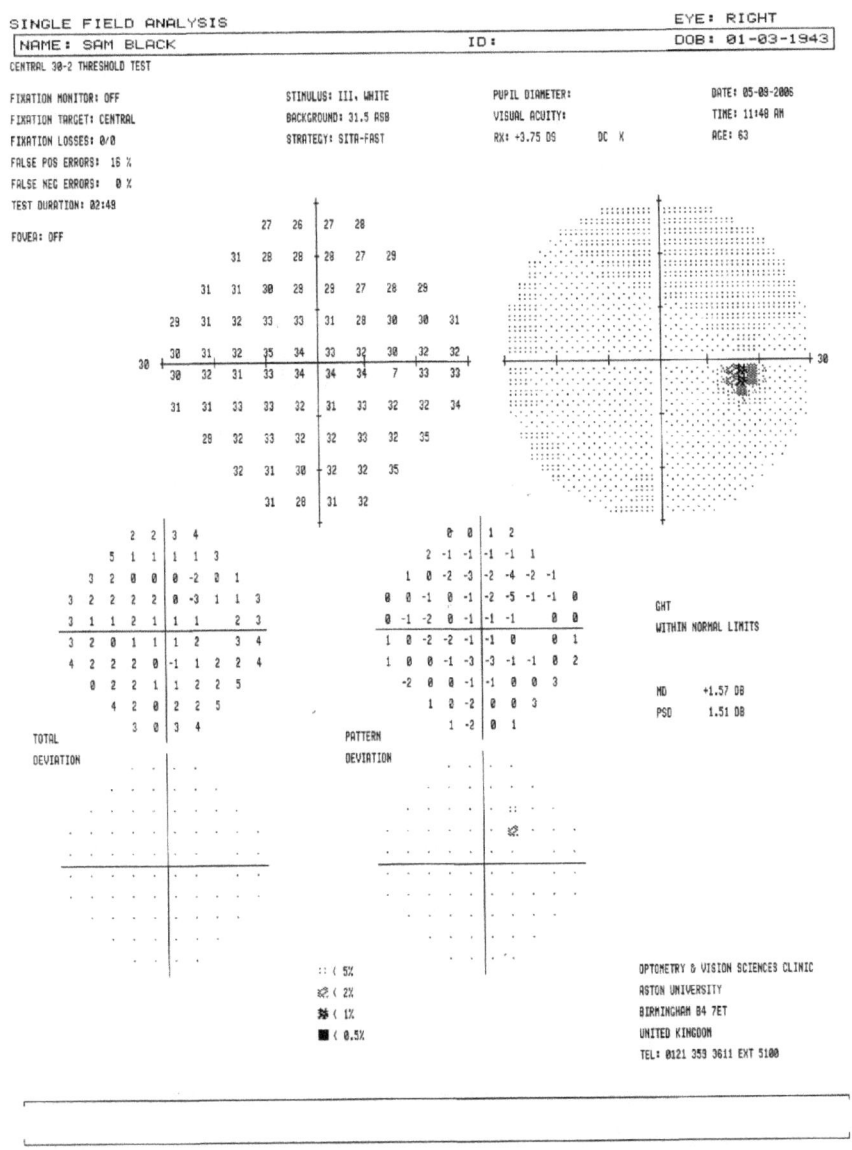

Figure 30 Humphrey plot depicting a normal visual field for the RE.

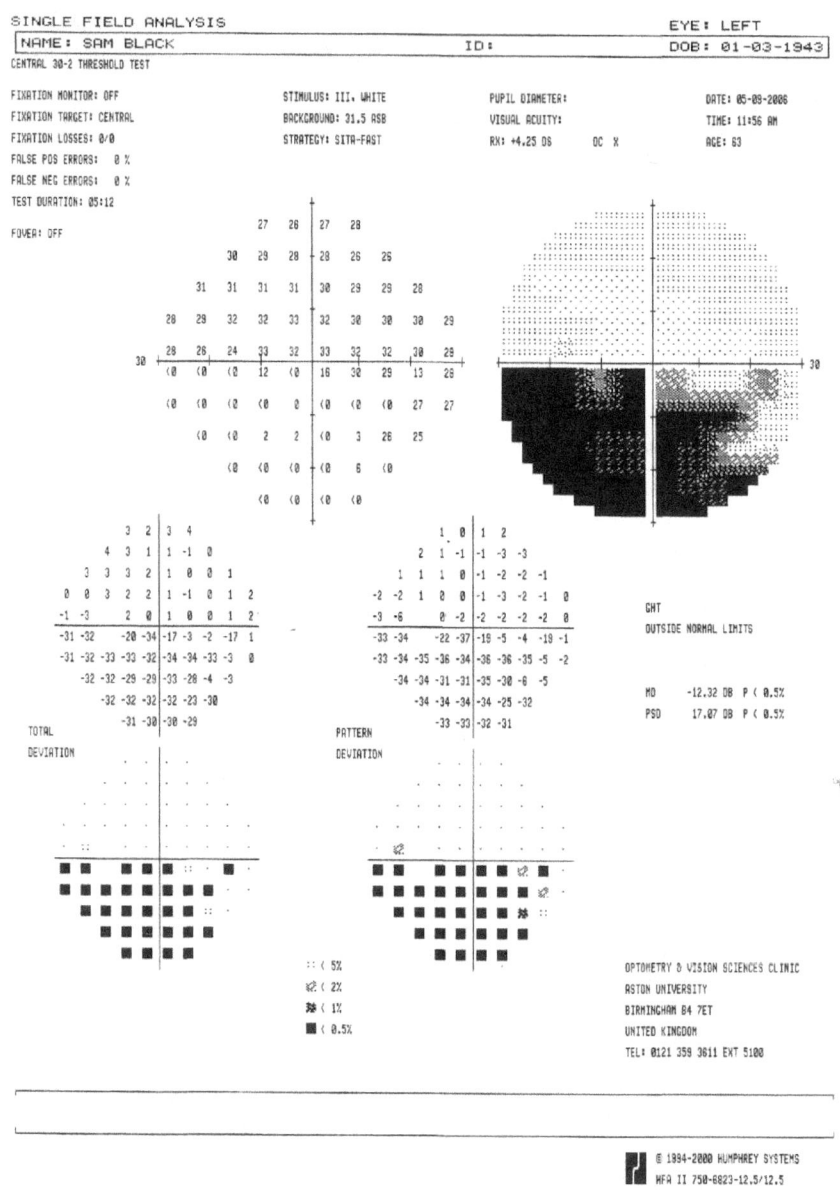

Figure 31 Humphrey plot depicting an inferior visual field defect in the LE.

Chapter 38 Gross perimetry-confrontation and peripheral fields

Introduction
Confrontation and peripheral fields are methods of making a speedy and gross assessment of a patient's visual field. Gross perimetry is an umbrella term for these two techniques. As with most visual field testing each eye is tested in turn. In confrontation the target is moved in a flat plane between the patient and practitioner, and the latter compares his/her monocular field with that of the patient. The target should be the same distance from the patient as it is from the practitioner and this is usually 25 cm. Peripheral fields involve moving the target in an arc centred on the patient's eye 33 cm from the patient. Peripheral fields analysis is the recommended technique as many practitioners find it difficult to bring the target from a position outside the normal visual field when working in a flat plane, due to shortness of the arms. It is essential to move from a position where the target is not seen to one where it is seen for both techniques.

A white spherical target, 5mm in diameter is recommended. However, if the background is pale (as it often is in the clinical environment) then a red spherical target three times the diameter of the white target i.e. 15 mm has to be used. The isopter for a 5/330 white target (5is the diameter of the target and 330 is the distance from the patient both in mm) closely follows the limits for the normal visual field, which are: 100 degrees temporally; 75 degrees inferiorly; 60 degrees nasally; 65 degrees superiorly.

It is occasionally useful to perform the test with a red target even when the background is not pale. For example, in chiasmal lesions due to pituitary tumours, colour desaturation occurs across the vertical midline. This modification to the technique will often enable far earlier diagnosis of a neurological lesion. An ideal target is a 15mm red hatpin, although some practitioners may use an object such as a coloured eyedropper to equally good effect, comparing the colour of the target in the four quadrants.

Use
The advantages of the above techniques are that they are quick and simple to perform, and in some circumstances may be the only way of making any visual field assessment; for example if the patient's co-operation is limited in the case of a cerebral vascular accident. The disadvantages are that these techniques are crude and the background against which they are conducted can vary. These techniques are purely qualitative and although suitable for identifying gross defects in the peripheral field, they are less than ideal for finer testing. For many high street

practices it may be the only way of assessing the visual field outside the central 25 degrees. In the main, if a defect is suspected using confrontation or peripheral fields, further investigation using more sophisticated instrumentation is indicated.

Procedure
In both techniques, the patient must cover one eye and fixate the examiner's opposite eye. The target has to be moved from a position where the patient initially cannot see it. The field plotted when the target is moved seeing to non-seeing is larger and when it is moved from non-seeing to seeing.

Confrontation
The target should be brought in from a position where the patient can't see it in a flat plane between the practitioner and the patient 25 cm from the patient and 25 cm from the practitioner.
Care must be taken to ensure that the target is exactly mid-way between examiner and subject.
In this technique the practitioner is comparing his/her field with that of the patient's.
The patient is asked to report when the target first appears.
When the patient fist sees the target continue moving it to the centre of the patient's visual field but not beyond.
Ask if the target disappears at any time when it is moved to the centre.
Repeat the procedure for 0, 45, 90, 135, 180, 225, 270, 315 and 360 meridians.

Peripheral fields
The target should be brought slowly from non-seeing to seeing round in an arc at 33 cm from the eye being tested.
The patient is asked to report when the target first appears.
When the patient fist sees the target continue moving it to the centre of the patient's visual field but not beyond.
Ask if the target disappears at any time when it is moved to the centre.
Repeat the procedure for 0, 45, 90, 135, 180, 225, 270, 315 and 360 meridians.

Recording findings
Gross perimetry is a qualitative procedure and therefore only subjective comments can be made on the results.

For example:
Confrontation visual fields full R&L to a 5/250 white target
R&L visual fields full to a 15/330 red target on peripheral fields testing

R&L temporal defect to a 15/250 red target on confrontation fields testing
L superior defect to a 5/330 white target on peripheral fields testing

Expected findings
Red 15 mm target field full to confrontation R and L.

White 5 mm target, peripheral and central fields full R and L.

Chapter 39 Henson Pro visual field analyser

Introduction
A Henson Pro is a bowl perimeter (radius 25 cm) that uses back projection LEDs as stimuli and is capable of testing the visual field out to an eccentricity of 72 degrees. The bowl luminance is maintained at 3.15 cd/m^2 (10asb). The perimeter is controlled from an external PC computer.

The Henson Pro has over 30 different test programs grouped into 5 different test strategies:

- Full Threshold
- Fast threshold
- Single stimulus supra-threshold
- Multiple stimulus supra-threshold
- Drivers.

Included in the software is a powerful database to which the visual field results can be stored and recalled.

Alignment of patient for testing
Position the patient on a chair in front of the Henson Pro such that the patient's brow touches the brow bar and the chin is on the chin rest. Adjust the chin rest so that the patient's eye level aligns with the marks on the Henson Pro.

Selecting a program
The Henson Pro offers four different strategies:

- Multiple stimulus supra-threshold
- Single stimulus supra-threshold
- Full threshold
- Drivers' tests (fixed intensity).

Choosing the program
For screening purposes select one of the supra-threshold strategies.
If speed is important the multiple stimulus supra-threshold strategy is approximately twice as fast as the single stimulus supra-threshold strategy for patients with little if any visual field defect.
If the patient has a known defect then the single stimulus strategy is considered to be a better option. In this situation the frequent failure of the patient to see all the stimuli in a multiple stimulus strategy results in repeated questioning that slows down the test and can lead to frustration for both the patient and the practitioner.

If the depth of a defect is required accurately a full threshold program should be used

If a large number of stimulus locations need to be tested a supra-threshold program should be chosen.

In order to quantify the extent of loss with the indices mean defect, loss variance and fluctuation use the full threshold strategy.

If a patient's suitability to drive a motor vehicle is required then use the Drivers Test.

Refractive correction

It is important for the patient to wear the correct refractive correction (suitable for a 25cm test distance) during the visual field test.

The Henson Pro is designed to be used with a special parametric lens set. This uses large diameter lenses that attach to a spectacle frame. This set overcomes the problem of lens rim artifacts, which are common when trial case lenses are used in tests that extend beyond the central 25 degrees.

Recommended additions (lens power to be added to the patients current distance prescription) are given in Table 4 below:

Patient Age (years)	Add on top of distance correction (DS)
40-44	+1.50
45-49	+2.00
+2.50	
55-59	+3.00
60-64	+3.50
>64	+4.00

Table 4 Add values according to patient age.

Supra-threshold tests

There are three supra-threshold tests incorporated within the Henson Pro:

- ➢ Central 25 degrees
- ➢ Full-field 60 degrees
- ➢ Armaly Central 30 degrees.

The first two can be run with the multiple or single stimulus strategy while the Armaly test can be run with the single stimulus strategy. Supra-threshold tests are ideal for rapid screening of the visual field but can also be used to monitor visual field loss. They present each stimulus at an intensity that is calculated to be above the patient's threshold by 5dB. If the patient sees the stimulus then it is assumed that no significant defect exists at the test location. If they fail to see the stimulus then it is presented a second time at the same intensity and if missed again presented at 8dB and then 12dB above the patient's threshold. This strategy takes into account the normal hill of vision. Peripheral stimuli being presented at a higher intensity than those in the centre of the visual field. This strategy is faster than the threshold strategies because, in a patient with no visual field each stimulus is presented only once. There are two different versions of the supra-threshold strategy provided with the Henson Pro software, multiple stimulus supra-threshold strategy and single stimulus supra-threshold strategy. Each strategy incorporates several different tests (central, full) and several levels of testing.

The supra-threshold phase of each test is preceded by a careful measurement of the threshold. This measurement is used to decide what the appropriate supra-threshold test intensity should be. Both tests have a number of different levels. In the central test these range from a quick 26-test point screening level test to one which tests 136 locations in extend mode. Both tests can be customised with the addition of extra stimulus locations.

Multiple stimulus supra-threshold test

The multiple stimulus supra-threshold tests each is composed of a pattern of 2, 3 or 4 stimuli. The patient responds to each presentation by telling the practitioner how many stimuli were seen. The use of multiple stimulus patterns makes the test approximately twice as fast as single stimulus tests.

The use of multiple stimulus test is semi-automated and requires more practitioner involvement than the single stimulus test. With a skilled perimetrist this can result in more reliable results with less variability. At the beginning of the test the perimetrist has to determine the patient's threshold. Stimuli are then presented at 5dB above this threshold estimate.

Single stimulus supra-threshold tests

Single stimulus supra-threshold tests are ideal for screening the visual field but can also be used monitor visual field loss. The test is fully automatic and requires no intervention by the practitioner other than to instruct the patient on what to do and to ensure that they have the correct refractive correction in front of the test eye and an occluder in front of the non-tested eye. It is a good idea to demonstrate to the patient.

Stimuli are presented one at a time, at an intensity calculated to be 5dB above a measurement of the patient's threshold. Stimuli that are not seen by the patient are presented a second time at the same intensity. If missed on both occasions the stimulus is marked as a miss and presented at 8dB above the threshold estimate. If missed at this intensity it will be presented at 12dB above the estimate. A grey scale indicates the depth of defect (5dB, 8dB or 12dB). The patient responds to each seen presentation by pressing their response button.

Procedure

Before starting the test you should ensure that the patient has the correct lens in front of the test eye and an occluder in front of the other eye.
The patient should then be instructed on what is involved and how they are to respond.
The patient's chin should be placed on the left side of the chin rest when testing the right eye and right side for the left eye.

The chin rest should be adjusted vertically until the eye is approximately in line with the markers on the side of the perimeter casing.

The first phase of the test finds the patient's threshold this is followed by the supra-threshold phase.

It is important to give clear and precise instructions to the patient at the outset and during the test.

A typical set of instructions is given below for both the multiple and single stimulus strategies.

Patient instructions for multiple stimulus
The test is going to take about two minutes. Make sure you are comfortable. Keep looking at the central red stimulus. Keep your eye as still as possible. The instrument will flash some lights to the side of where you are looking. Each flash will be of 2, 3 or 4 lights. I want you, after each flash to tell me the number of lights you saw. To begin with the lights will be fairly bright. They will then get dimmer and dimmer until you cannot see them. Do not guess-if you are not sure you saw any lights say none.

When performing the supra-threshold phase of the test: The lights will be brighter now. Continue to look at the central red light. Just tell me the number of lights that you see in each flash. I may ask you to tell me where the lights you saw were.

Patient instructions for single stimulus
The test is going to take about two minutes. Make sure you are comfortable. Press the response key when you see a stimulus. You will not see all the lights. Do not guess. If you are not sure you saw a light do not press the button. Keep looking at the central red stimulus. Keep your eye as still as possible. If you want to take a break hold down the response key. I will start with a demonstration of the test. When you are comfortable with what is required I will start the test.

Establishing the threshold at the onset of a supra-threshold test
At the onset of a supra-threshold test it is necessary to obtain an estimate of the patient's threshold. This estimate is used to calculate the test intensity, which is set at 5dB above the threshold estimate. See table 74.0 for typical threshold levels.

Single stimulus strategy
In the single stimulus supra-threshold strategy this is done automatically. At four locations, one in each quadrant, the threshold is determined with a full threshold strategy. The second most sensitive location is then taken as the threshold estimate from which the supra-threshold intensity is calculated. Once the threshold has been established the Henson Pro will automatically proceed to the supra-threshold phase of the examination. The rate at which the stimuli are presented can be adjusted at any stage of the examination by clicking the right and left arrows at the end of Presentation Rate Scale or by pressing the left or right arrow in the keyboard. The test can be suspended at any time by clicking over the stop button.

Multiple stimulus strategy
In the multiple stimulus strategy the threshold is determined via a pre-programmed series presentations. After each presentation the patient, who needs to be carefully instructed, reports back to the perimetrist whether or not they saw any of the stimuli and the perimetrist feeds this information back into the program.

Patterns are presented by clicking over the present button or pressing the keyboard space bar. The practitioner can present the stimuli as many times as they like. If the patient reports that they saw some of the stimuli then the practitioner should enter this response by clicking over the yes button or pressing the keyboard Y key. If the patient reports they did not see any of the stimuli then the practitioner should enter this response by clicking over the No button or pressing the keyboard N key. Once the threshold has been established the Henson Pro will automatically proceed to the supra-threshold phase of the examination.

Typical threshold sensitivity levels
The table below gives typical values for the threshold levels. While individual patients are likely to differ from these values, large unexplainable departures (>3 dB should be viewed with caution). The perimetrist should question whether or not the patient fully understood the instructions. In these instances it wise to repeat the instructions and the demonstrating phase. Click over the 'Start Eye Again' option Under the File menu bar option. See Table 5 for typical threshold levels for the Henson Pro.

Age (years)	Threshold Sensitivity (dB)
<40	38 - 40
41 – 50	37 - 39
51 - 60	36 - 38
61 - 70	35 - 37
71 – 80	34 - 36

Table 5 Typical threshold levels for the Henson Pro.

Intensity changes in multiple stimulus tests
The Henson Pro starts off its testing phase at 5dB above the threshold estimate. Stimuli missed twice at this increment should be presented at higher increments in order to measure the depth of the defect. There are 3 different supra-threshold test increments, 5dB, 8dB and 12dB.

Each of the test intensities has a button on the icon bar and the button that appears to be down gives the currently selected increment. To switch to a different intensity click over the appropriate button. The intensity can also be changed by pressing the up and down arrow keys and by selecting intensity from the menu bar and clicking over the desired value.

Missed stimuli in multiple stimulus test
It is not unusual for a patient with no visual field loss to miss the occasional stimulus. To differentiate these and misses due to genuine field loss the pattern should be presented a second time and only if the patient again reports an incorrect number of stimuli should the perimetrist proceed to establish which stimuli were missed and to enter their locations.

To establish which stimuli were missed the perimetrist needs to asks the patient where they saw stimuli. It is often helpful at this stage to tell the patient to consider the bowl as a clock face and to give the hour positions of the stimuli. Once you have established which stimuli were missed place the pointer over each and press the right mouse button. To correct mistakes, i.e. remove missed stimuli, place the pointer over the stimulus and double click the right mouse button. Stimuli missed at a 5dB increment should be tested at higher intensities.

Extend
All the test programs in the Henson Pro can be extended. Each program starts off with a basic test. In the central supra-threshold strategy this would test 26 test points. At the end of this test the perimetrist can opt to increase the number of test locations to 68 (a second extension can take it to 136). To extend the test click the pointer either over the Red Cross Extend icon or at the Options menu button then Extend. The red-cross extend icon disappears after two extensions.

The extend facility means that the perimetrist does not have to decide upon the extent of the test before they have collected any data. This improves efficiency in two ways. The perimetrist is not locked in to an extensive test when it is clear, well before the end, that further testing is not going to add information. When it is decided that a more extensive test is needed the perimetrist does not have to repeat a large number of measurements.

The mouse can be used to add test locations or correct existing ones. This facility is useful for checking the result from a particular location or removing artefactual data such as that produced by a correcting lens rim. This can be done either during the test or at the end of the test. The action of the mouse buttons differ for threshold and supra-threshold tests and the instructions below apply to supra-threshold tests only.

To add a new test location or to re-test an already tested location place the mouse pointer over the location you want to present the stimulus and press the left mouse button. The test intensity is represented by the selected intensity icon (the one that appears to be down) on the icon bar. To change this simply click over the desired intensity (5dB, 8dB or 12dB). To enter a location as missed, place the pointer over the location and press the right mouse button. To correct a test location marked with a missed pattern. Place the pointer over the location and double click the right button.

Intensity changes in single stimulus supra-threshold tests.
The intensity is adjusted automatically during the single stimulus supra-threshold test. If a stimulus is missed the program will come back to the location and re-test it at the same intensity. If it is missed a second time it will mark it as a missed location (5dB) and come back to test it at a higher intensity. It will repeat this until either the stimulus is seen or not seen at the highest intensity level (12dB). There are 3 different supra-threshold test increments, 6dB, 8dB and 12dB. Each of the test intensities has a button on the icon bar and the button that appears to be down gives the currently selected increment.

Recording findings
See Figures 32 and 33 for Henson Pro plots depicting R and L superior visual field defects (quadrantopia), respectively.

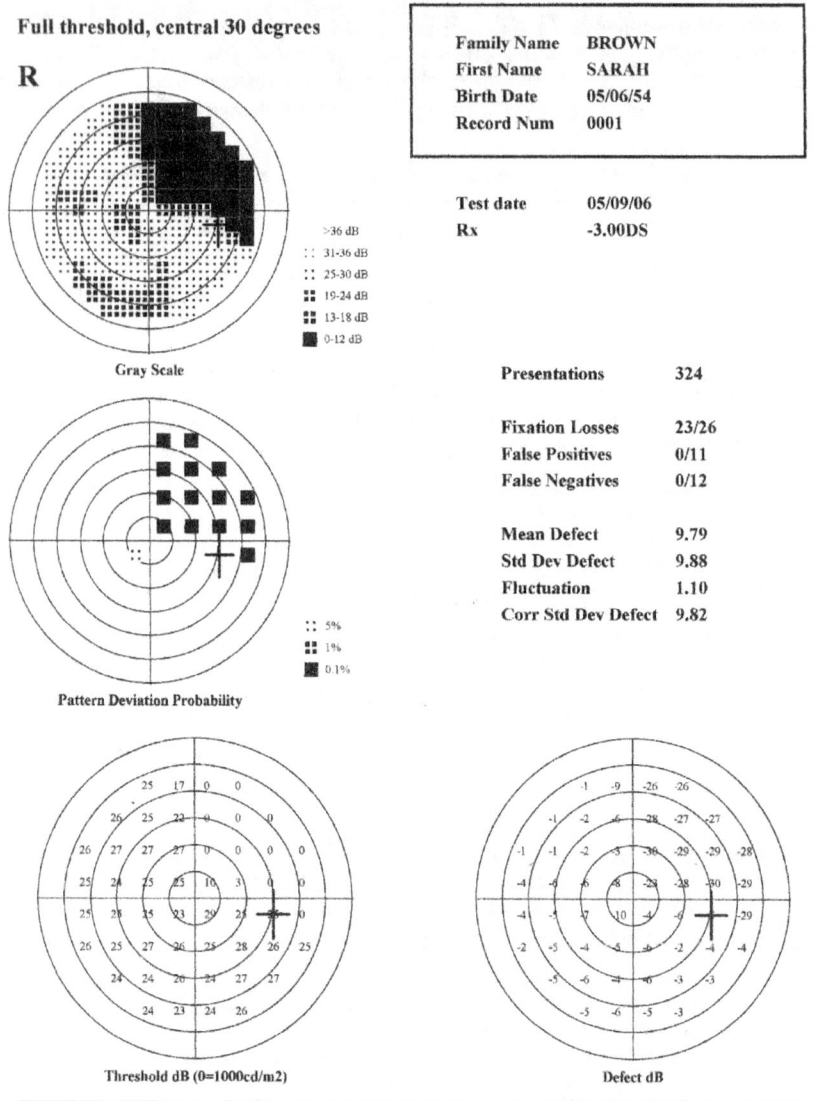

Figure 32 right eye superior quadrantopia.

Art of Clinical Practice in Optometry

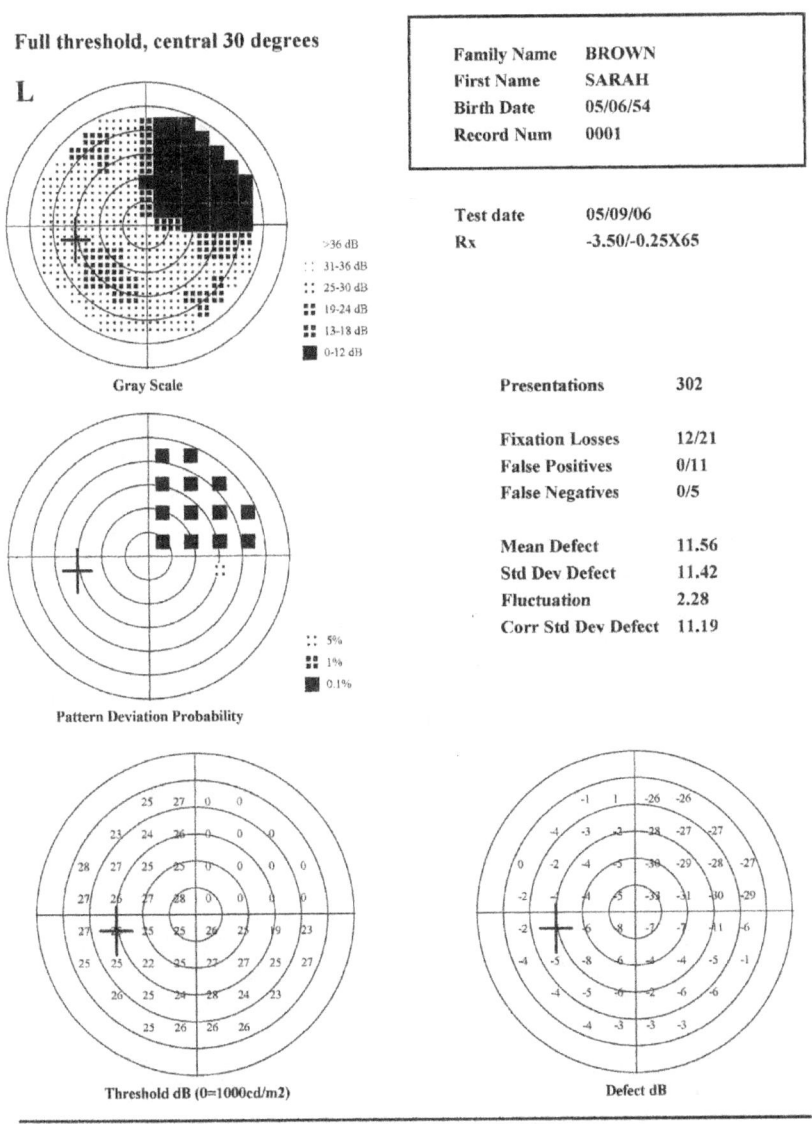

Figure 33 left eye superior quadrantopia.

Chapter 40 Ishihara colour vision test

Introduction
The Ishihara test consists of a series of plates designed to provide a quick and accurate assessment of colour vision deficiency of congenital origin. Most cases are characterised by a red or green deficiency.

Use
Screening for congenital or acquired red or green colour vision deficiency.

Procedure
Fluorescent room lights should be turned on but all light sources using tungsten filament lamps should be off as this type of illumination can make the test easier to pass for someone with a mild red colour vision deficiency.
Plates should be held 75 cm from the subject and tilted so that the plane of the plate is at right angles to the line of vision.
Each plate should be identified within three seconds.
For those patients unable to read numerals, those plates near the end of the book with winding lines between two Xs should be used. Lines should be traced with a brush in less than ten seconds.
Make a note of whether any plates were identified incorrectly.
If any of the screening plates are incorrectly identified ask the observer to identify the classification plates.
Mark the results on the Ishihara score sheet.

Hints and tips
When testing for congenital colour deficiency it is appropriate for the patient to carry out the test with both eyes open.
When an acquired colour vision defect is suspected the test should be conducted monocularly.

Recording findings
The score sheet can be used to determine the type of deficiency by noting which plates have been identified incorrectly.

Expected findings
All numbers identified correctly.

Chapter 41 City University colour vision test

Introduction
The City University test comprises selected paper colour samples, which must not be touched. On each page, four colour samples surround a central spot and the subject must choose the one that most closely resembles the colour of the central spot. Each page provides the opportunity for a normal response-the patient identifies the normal spot as being the one that is identical in colour, or is most nearly similar in colour to the central spot. Each page provides possible protan, deutan or tritan confusions that may be mixed with a normal response since some observers may find more than one near match on a page. A consistent regime must be used, taking care to illuminate the test correctly.

Use
Screening for congenital and all types of acquired colour vision deficiency.

Procedure
Fluorescent room lights should be turned on but all light sources using tungsten filament lamps should be off as this type of illumination can make the test easier to pass for someone with a mild red colour vision deficiency
Hold the booklet at 35 cm from the patient with the pages at right angles to the line of sight
Show the demonstration page 'A' and say: Here are four coloured spots surrounding one in the centre. Tell me which spot looks most near in colour to the one in the centre. Use the words top, bottom, right or left. Please do not touch the pages.
Show the test plates 1 to 10 in turn
Allow about 3 seconds for each page
The plates are divided into six chroma 4 and four chroma 2 plates (smaller spots).

Recording findings
The test can be scored by noting the response on the score sheet and then determining if the response is normal or abnormal.

Expected findings
All matching stimuli correctly identified.

Hints and tips
When testing for congenital colour deficiency it is appropriate for the patient to carry out the test with both eyes open.
When an acquired colour vision defect is suspected the test should be conducted monocularly.

Chapter 42 Amsler grid

Introduction
The Amsler grid is a test chart used to determine quality of central vision and allows the analysis of disturbances of visual function, which accompany the beginning and evolution of maculopathies. The standard chart to be used in this practical consists of a square with white lines on a black background in which horizontal and vertical parallel lines make up a perfectly squared surface. In the centre is a white spot that serves as the fixation point.

Use
This test is useful for those patients that complain of central field loss and/or distorted central vision.

Procedure
The chart should be used at a distance of 30cms, be evenly illuminated with the patient wearing any required refractive correction.
Ophthalmoscopy should not be performed directly before this test.
Explain to the patient 'Fix your gaze on the central dark spot and at the same time observe the whole chart and the details of the network'.
The Amsler grid manual recommends the use of six questions presented in a logical order to determine the presence of any sensorial dysfunction.

Six patient questions
1. Do you see the white spot in the centre of the square?
2. Keeping the gaze fixed upon the white spot in the centre, can you see the four corners of the big square? Can you also see the four sides of the square? In other words can you see the whole of the square?
3. While always keeping the gaze fixed on the central fixation point, do you see the network intact, in the whole square? Or are there interruptions in the network of squares, like holes or spots. Is it blurred in any place? And if so, where?
4. Always keeping the gaze fixed on the white spot in the centre do you see all the lines, both horizontal and vertical, quite straight and parallel? In other words, is every small square equal in size and perfectly regular?
5. Always fixing the gaze upon the centre point, independently of blurred spots and distortions, can you see anything else? A movement of certain lines? A vibration or wavering? Anything shining? A colour or tint? And if so, where on the square?
6. Keeping the central point fixed at what distance from this point do you place the blur or distortion you see? How many small intact squares do you find between the blur or distortion and the central point you are keeping your gaze upon? This last question may not be relevant in this practical.

Art of Clinical Practice in Optometry

Note any observations the patient makes and if there are any visual disturbances try and locate them on the grid by asking the subject to draw them on the recording chart. This looks the same as the testing grid but has a black grid on a white background.

Hints and tips
Use the white grid on a black background version of the Amsler grid as the standard test.
Using the black grid on white background record card as the test stimulus should be avoided.
Some patients experience visual distortions unconnected to ocular disease when viewing such a stimulus and the patient could incorrectly be diagnosed as having a macular problem.
Encourage the patient to fix the central spot.

Recording findings
See Figure 34 for an example of metamorphopsia and Figure 35 for an example of a central scotoma as detected using the Amsler grid.

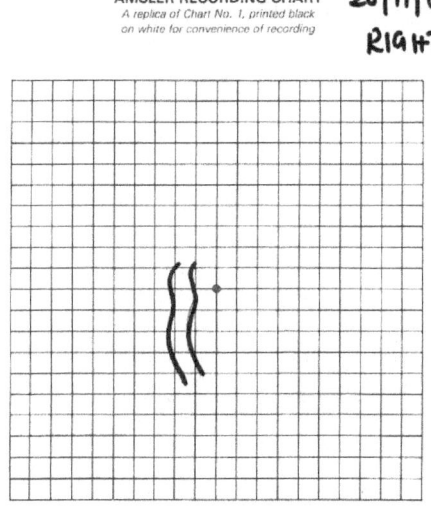

Figure 34 Metamorphopsia detected using the Amsler grid

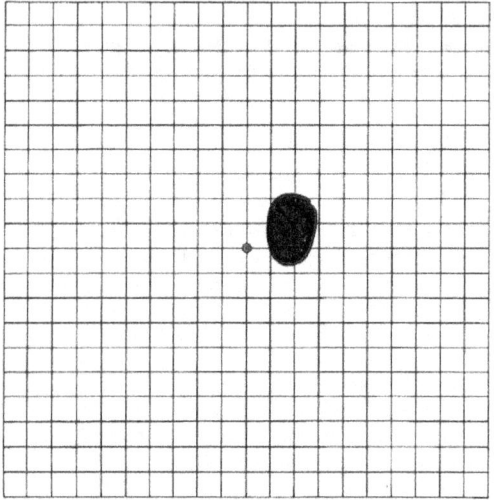

Figure 35 Central scotoma detected using the Amsler grid

Chapter 43 Pelli-Robson contrast threshold chart

Introduction
The letters on the Pelli-Robson contrast threshold chart are organised into groups of three i.e. triplets, with two triplets per line. Within each triplet all letters have the same contrast and the contrast decreases from one triplet to the next while the letter size stays constant throughout the chart (roughly equivalent to a 6/60 letter). In each set there are two charts with a different arrangement of letters so that learning effects can be kept to a minimum when testing monocularly and binocularly. See Figure 36.

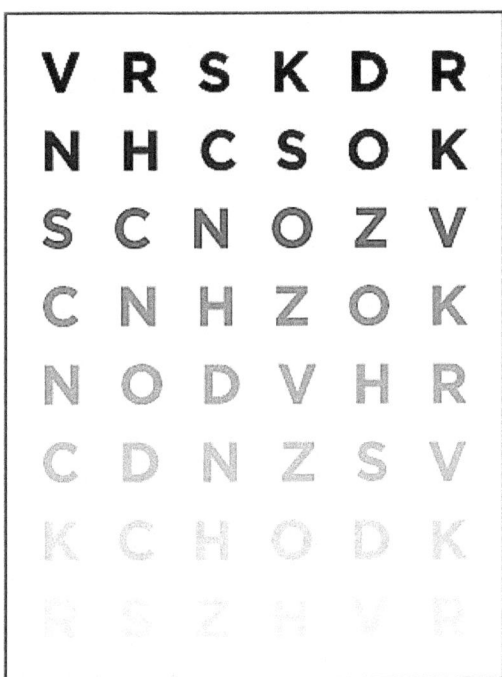

Figure 36 Pelli-Robson contrast threshold chart.

Use
Contrast sensitivity testing using the Pelli-Robson chart is useful for those patients who have problems with their everyday functional vision but have good levels of VA. This clinical scenario sometimes arises with certain types of cataract.

Procedure
Position the patient 1m from the chart.
Appropriate refractive correction should be worn for this working distance.
The patient should wear their normal refractive correction for distance.
If they are presbyopic they should view the chart through a +1D lens.
A Halberg clip is useful for this purpose.
Occlude one eye.
Ask the patient to read from top left to as far down the chart as possible.
Instruct the patient to guess even when they believe the letters are invisible.
Allow 20 seconds for the faintest letters near the patient's threshold.
Score miss-called Cs, Os or Ds as correct i.e. if the observer calls a C as an O count it as correct, the same if they call a D as a C and so on.
Research has shown that a more accurate result is obtained when this scoring method is used.
Repeat for LE and again with both eyes open.

Hints and tips
Each correct letter has a contrast threshold value of 0.05 log units.
Scoring in terms of log units is reserved for research.
A more clinical approach is to score in terms of contrast percentage.

Recording findings
Pelli-Robson chart RE 44% LE 2.8% Both 3.9%.

Expected findings
Young patient without ocular disease RE 2.8% LE 2.8% Both 1.9%.
Old patient without ocular disease RE 3.9% LE 3.9% Both 2.8%.

Chapter 44 Modified monocular indirect ophthalmoscopy

Introduction
A thorough fundus examination is important and required in all young patients with strabismus or amblyopia in order to rule out organic causes of amblyopia prior to the initiation of treatment. Examination of very young children can be difficult especially when a detailed view of the macula and optic nerve is required. The magnification and patient co-operation obtained with head mounted binocular indirect ophthalmoscopy using a 20D lens, and slit lamp biomicroscopy using a 90D or other similar lens means that fundus examination is usually difficult or impossible on younger children. Also the magnification may be inadequate to allow accurate evaluation of posterior pole details. The direct ophthalmoscope is often the best available instrument for detailed retinal examination in young patients.

However, children often become frightened as the examiner approaches closely, as is necessary with the direct ophthalmoscope and co-operation is lost. Additionally, children often fix the ophthalmoscope light and track it as the examiner moves it, allowing examination of the macula but not of the disc. The field of view is small and the magnification is more than is usually necessary. This will prevent the examiner from seeing the 'big picture'.

To avoid these difficulties the direct ophthalmoscope can be used in conjunction with a 20D condensing lens, the type used with head mounted binocular indirect ophthalmoscopes. This combination provides a moderately magnified and wider angle, view of the posterior pole and avoids the close proximity between the patient and examiner required when using a direct ophthalmoscope alone. The technique has been noted for providing a good view of the retina through a small pupil when dilation is contraindicated.

Use
This technique can be used for the ocular examination of young children. The equipment that is required is:
Standard hand held direct ophthalmoscope.
Variety of plus powered condensing lenses; +20D, +28D, +30D and 2.2 Panretinal.
Dilating agents (0.5% or 1.0% tropicamide).

Procedure
To begin the examination visualise a red reflex through the direct ophthalmoscope when held approximately 18 cm from the patient's eye.

Place a +20D condensing lens 3 to 5 cm in front of the patient's eye in the path of the direct ophthalmoscope light beam.

Move slightly toward or away from the patient until a clear image of the retina is observed.

An inverted, aerial image of the retina is produced, located between the observer and the lens.

The apparent magnification will gradually increase as the examiner moves closer to this image (that is, closer to the patient), allowing more detailed examination.

A magnification of 4 to 5X is obtained by moving closer to the image.

As the examiner moves closer additional lenses in the ophthalmoscope are needed, to keep the image clear depending on the accommodative needs of the examiner.

Experience has shown that a viewing distance of approximately 18 cm from the patient is optimal, providing suitable magnification and a wide field of view.

Hints and tips

Lateral movement and rotation of the direct ophthalmoscope during the examination gives good parallax clues to depth and helps to partially overcome the lack of stereoacuity with this monocular technique.

Lateral and longitudinal adjustments of the lens may be made to optimise the field of view.

When viewing finer fundus details increase the lamp intensity and magnification

The retina can be explored by moving the lens and the slit horizontally and vertically in the same direction.

The amount of pupil dilation will limit the area of retina that can be explored this way.

More peripheral retina can be explored by asking the patient to fix in the cardinal positions of gaze and repositioning the lens and slit beam accordingly.

Recording findings

Vitreous – floaters.
Neural retinal rim – pale nasal quadrant.
Disc margins – poorly defined.
Cup to disc ratio – value of ratio.
Crescents – choroidal.
Disc anomalies/abnormalities – tilting.
Vessels – tortuosity.
Fundus – pigmented.
Macula – haemorrhage.

Expected findings

Vitreous – clear.
Neural retinal rim – pink.
Disc margins – well defined.
Cup to disc ratio – (value of ratio).
Crescents – none, choroidal, scleral.
Disc anomalies/abnormalities – none.
Vessels – ¾ artery to vein ratio.
Fundus – healthy.
Macula – foveal reflex present.

Chapter 45 Head mounted indirect ophthalmoscopy

Introduction
Binocular indirect ophthalmoscopy (BIO) is a technique used to evaluate the entire ocular fundus. It allows stereoscopic, wide-angled, high-resolution views of the entire fundus and overlying vitreous. Its optical principles and illumination options allow for visualisation of the fundus regardless of high ametropia, hazy ocular media, or central opacities.

Light beams directed into the patient's eye produce reflected observation beams from the retina. These beams are focused to a viewable, aerial image following placement of a high plus-powered condensing lens at its focal distance in front of the patient's eye. The resultant image is real, magnified, reversed left to right, inverted top to bottom and located between the examiner and the condensing lens. The observer views this image through the oculars of the head-borne indirect ophthalmoscope.

Use
Stereoscopic examination of the vitreous and retina.
The equipment needed for this technique is:
Head band for comfortable instrument placement.
Light source with variable intensity illumination beams directed downward and reflected laterally by an adjustable mirrored surface in the main housing.
Knobs to align the low plus powered eyepieces (+2.00 to +2.50 D) with the examiners inter-pupillary distance.
Variety of plus powered condensing lenses; +20D. +28D, +30D and 2.2 Panretinal.
Dilating agents (0.5% or 1.0% tropicamide-for maximum dilation used in conjunction with 2.5% phenylephrine).

Procedure
Head mounted BIO adjustment
Place the loose BIO onto the head and position the bottom of the front headband one index finger width above the eyebrows.
Tighten the crown strap until this headband position begins to stabilise.
Position the back head strap on or below the occipital notch and tighten until secure.
Loosen the knobs that control the instruments main housing (oculars and light tower).
Fixing straight ahead and level, vertically position the oculars to within eye lash distance from the observers eyes aligned tangential to or slightly angled downward

from the ocular surface; this should maximise the visual field and minimise horizontal diplopia.
Horizontally align each ocular by closing one eye and fixating a centrally positioned thumb at 40 to 50 cm.
Adjust the ocular alignment knob or slide the oculars to place an identical centrally positioned thumb in each ocular's field of view.
Turn on the light source and fixate straight ahead on a wall at 40 to 50 cm looking at the projected light source.
Use the mirror knob to vertically place the light source at the upper one-half to one-third of the field.

Head mounted BIO technique
Best with dilated pupils.
Headset in place, set the voltage to mid-range.
Hold a +20 D condensing lens with the thumb, index, and middle fingers of the right hand.
The more convex surface should be toward the observer and the white-ringed edge closest to the patient.
From a working distance of 18 to 20 inches, direct the light beam into the pupil, producing a complete red pupillary reflex.
Pull backward on the lens, maintaining the central position of the pupil reflex, until the entire lens fills with the fundus image.
Make fine adjustments in the lens tilt and vertex distance to produce a distortion-free full lens view.

Hints and tips
Take time to set up this instrument as poor eye piece alignment may result in diplopia.
Warn the patient that the light will be bright.
Wait until the patient is well dilate before starting the examination.

Recording findings
Vitreous – floaters.
Neural retinal rim – pale nasal quadrant.
Disc margins – poorly defined.
Cup to disc ratio – value of ratio.
Crescents – choroidal.
Disc anomalies/abnormalities – tilting.
Vessels – tortuosity.
Fundus – pigmented.
Macula – haemorrhage.

Expected findings
Vitreous – clear.
Neural retinal rim – pink.
Disc margins – well defined.
Cup to disc ratio – (value of ratio).
Crescents – none, choroidal, scleral.

Disc anomalies/abnormalities – none.
Vessels – ¾ artery to vein ratio.
Fundus – healthy.
Macula – foveal reflex present.

Chapter 46 Slit lamp biomicroscopy

Introduction
A non-contact auxiliary condensing lens is used in conjunction with the slit lamp to provide an inverted, wide field, stereoscopic image with good resolution. The technique is often referred to as slit lamp BIO (binocular indirect ophthalmoscopy).

Use
This technique can be used to evaluate the health of the posterior segment of the eye and in particular to detect the presence of macular oedema. Views out to the peripheral retina may be obtained with some lenses and a well dilated pupil. This is useful in order to determine the presence of retinal neovascularisation, tears and features that pre-dispose the retina to detachment.

The equipment required for this technique is:
- Numerous condensing lenses are available; they are plus powered with two convex aspheric surfaces. See Table 2.
- +60D version has the greatest magnification and is best used for the disc and macula.
- +78D version is a good general diagnostic lens.
- +90D is useful with small pupils, as is the SuperPupil.
- +66D produces a high definition view of the disc and the macular.
- SuperField, which is approximately +90D, is a good all-rounder.
- They are available in clear or blue-free, 'yellow retina protector glass'.
- This is considered to be more comfortable for the patient and minimises the risk of phototoxic retinal damage due to prolonged exposure to the focussed beam.
- An +81D lens is also available which provides a view similar to that of a +78D when held one way round, and a view similar to that produced by a +90D lens when held the other way round.
- Slit lamp
- Dilating agents, 0.5% or 1.0% tropicamide and 2.5% phenylephrine.

Table 6 Main characteristics of positive condensing lenses used with the slit lamp

Lens Size	Diameter (mm)	Magnification	Field of view (degrees)	Working distance (mm)
60D	31	1.09	67	11.0
78D	31	0.87	73	7.0
90D	21.5	0.72	69	6.5
SuperField	26	0.71	120	6.0 - 6.5

Actual magnification of ocular structures is determined by the magnification of the slit lamp eye piece lenses e.g. the SuperField will provide 7.1x magnification if used with 10x eye piece lenses

Slit lamp set up
- Click stop in
- Beam straight ahead
- 2 to 3 mm beam width
- Maximum beam height
- No filter
- Medium illumination
- 10 to 15X magnification.

Procedure
Minimal lamp intensity should be used in a darkened room.
Select a condensing lens.
Ensure that the condensing lens surfaces are clean.
Hold the lens vertically between the thumb and index finger of the left hand to examine the patient's right eye.
Hold the lens in the right hand to examine the patient's left eye.
Some lenses may be used with a lens holder mounted on the upright support of the headrest or an adapter that rests against the patient's eyelids; these accessories may make fundus observation easier for the novice.
Instruct the patient to fixate straight ahead, to stare wide and to blink normally.
Centre the beam in the patient's right pupil and focus on the cornea.
Place the lens in front of the patient's eye, directly in front of the cornea so the back surface just clears the lashes (approximately 11 mm for the +60D, 7 mm for the +78D, and 6.5 mm for the +90D and the SuperField NC from the patient's cornea).
These condensing lenses can be used either way round.
Avoid touching the patient's eyelashes if possible.
Lens positioning may be made easier by placing the other fingers on the brow bar or the patient's forehead.
When the lens is properly positioned, a blurred red fundus reflex will appear when looking through the oculars of the slit lamp.
Use the joystick to focus on the fundus image by slowly moving away from the cornea, keeping the beam centred in the pupil.
When scratches on the surface of the condensing lens come into view the slit lamp needs to be pulled back a little more (about 1 cm) for the retina to be in focus.
Once the retinal image is focussed, widen the beam to observe a greater area of the fundus.
The magnification can be changed to a higher setting at this time.
Scan across the entire lens.
At this stage keep the lens still.
In order to view the peripheral retina ask the patient to change fixation into the nine cardinal positions of gaze.
It will be necessary to realign the lens and refocus the slit lamp.

To reduce interfering reflections, tilt the lens or increase the setting of the illumination arm to 10 degrees nasal or temporal once the fundus has been located and focussed.

Depending upon the design of the slit lamp, a +60D or a +78D lens may require the patient to move away from the headrest slightly in order to be able to focus the retina.

Centre the slit lamp beam in the left eye and repeat steps 3 through 6 on the patient's left eye.

Hints and tips
Lateral and longitudinal adjustments of the lens may be made to optimise the field of view.
When viewing finer fundus details increase the lamp intensity and magnification.
The retina can be explored by moving the lens and the slit horizontally and vertically in the same direction.
The amount of pupil dilation will limit the area of retina that can be explored this way. More peripheral retina can be explored by asking the patient to fix in the cardinal positions of gaze and repositioning the lens and slit beam accordingly.

Recording findings
Vitreous – floaters.
Neural retinal rim – pale nasal quadrant.
Disc margins – poorly defined.
Cup to disc ratio – value of ratio.
Crescents – choroidal.
Disc anomalies/abnormalities – tilting.
Vessels – tortuosity.
Fundus – pigmented.
Macula – haemorrhage.

Expected findings
Vitreous – clear.
Neural retinal rim – pink.
Disc margins – well defined.
Cup to disc ratio – (value of ratio).
Crescents – none, choroidal, scleral.
Disc anomalies/abnormalities – none.
Vessels – ¾ artery to vein ratio.
Fundus – healthy.
Macula – foveal reflex present.

Chapter 47 Slit-lamp ophthalmoscopy with negative lenses

Introduction
Negative powered auxiliary lenses in conjunction the slit-lamp biomicroscope can be used to view the vitreous and retina and in particular the optic nerve head and the macula. For practitioners with some level of binocularity a binocular direct image is viewed.

Use
The use of the slit-lamp biomicroscope allows a stereoscopic view of the retina which is useful in assessing the elevation of interesting features. The auxiliary lenses provide high magnification with excellent resolution. Many practitioners experienced with this procedure suggest that it surpasses a 78 or 90D indirect examination in detecting subtle abnormalities. Although several aspects of this type of procedure prevent it from becoming part of a routine examination, there is no other way to achieve a comparable sense of depth.

Slit-lamp direct ophthalmoscopy can be performed with several types of auxiliary lens. The types that will be discussed here are the non-contact Hruby lens (-55D) and two types of diagnostic contact lens. All lenses have a high minus power which produces an upright virtual image which is not laterally reversed. Contact lenses also have an advantage in that the examiner's view of the retina is not interrupted by the patient's blink reflex, although the use of contact lenses with this technique is contraindicated in those situations where the minimal trauma associated with the technique would be harmful to the patient, such as, the period immediately following an eye operation, if there is any active corneal disease, the presence of a penetrating or perforating injury and before other ocular procedures that depend on corneal clarity e.g. fundus photography. Advantages of this technique are high magnification and a stereoscopic view. The main disadvantage is the small field of view.

Slit lamp set up
- Click stop in
- Beam straight ahead
- 2 mm beam width
- Maximum beam height
- No filter
- Medium illumination
- 10 to 15X magnification.

Procedure
Diagnostic contact lens
Scan the anterior eye with the biomicroscope to rule out conditions that preclude use of this procedure.
Instil topical anaesthetic.
Fill the concave surface of the lens with coupling solution.
Hold the lens with the thumb and first finger of your dominant hand such that it can easily be applied to the patient's eye.
Move the slit lamp in front of the eye that is not being examined to allow easier access.
Ask the patient to look down, and retract their upper lid with the thumb of your non-dominant hand.
As the patient to look down and then place the lower rim of the lens into the patient's lower conjunctival sac.
Tilt the lens to contact the cornea and then slowly release the upper lid. Maintain light pressure on the lens to prevent the patient's blinking from dislodging it.
Look around the side of the instrument and position the slit lamp beam in the centre of the lens.
Looking through the oculars, you should be able to see a red reflex.
Push the slit lamp gently towards the patient; any opacities in the lens or vitreous should become apparent.
Once the retina is in focus, the area under observation can be altered by changing the patient's fixation with the slit lamp fixation target.
The slit lamp must be moved horizontally and vertically to keep the slit beam in line with the pupil.
The magnification and beam width can be altered to improve the view, although be aware that this may become uncomfortable for the patient.
Remove the contact lens when the examination is finished. You may need to apply light pressure to the globe in order to release the suction from the lens, or alternatively ask the patient to look up and blink.
Irrigate any excess coupling solution using sterile saline.
Use fluorescein to check for corneal staining.

Non-contact lens examination
The procedure is exactly the same as for the contact lens, except that there is no need to use a coupling gel as the auxiliary lens (Hruby lens) is held in front of the eye, as close as possible to the cornea without touching the lashes.

Hints and tips
When using a contact lens make sure that there are no bubbles in the coupling gel as these will obscure the view.
Artificial tears may need to be recommended for 12 to 24 hours following the procedure as it may induce superficial corneal staining.
Mirrored lens examination should be performed at the end of routine eye examination; otherwise results may be contaminated.

Intraocular pressure is reduced because some aqueous humour is forced out through the drainage channels by the pressure exerted on the globe.
The cornea is slightly hazy from the topical anaesthetic, viscous coupling gel and microtrauma from the lens.
This blurs the patient's vision rendering any subjective examination results invalid.
The examiners view inward is also compromised affecting other types of ophthalmoscopy.
It is important to remember that the view through the mirrors is reversed; descriptions and illustrations should be anatomically correct.
For retinal evaluation it is necessary to indicate where the lesion is located on the retina, not where it appears to be through the mirror.
The mirrored lens must be constantly held in contact with the patient's eye
The lens can be rotated and angled to enhance the view.
The slit beam should be kept perpendicular to mirror as the lens is rotated.
The examination may be long and the arm supporting the lens may become fatigued.
An elbow rest such as a tissue box placed on the slit lamp table can support the arm and make the examiner more comfortable.
Reduce interference from reflections on the Hruby lens by tilting is slightly.
The image is upright and not laterally reversed which aids in interpretation and record keeping.
The patient is allowed to blink and the view of the retina will not be interrupted, as the lids do not pass between the lens and the eye.
It is acceptable to manoeuvre the lens by changing its angle in order to enhance the view.
High magnification will reduce the field of view and any hand tremor may be exacerbated.
Because the posterior pole is under examination the patient may find it very uncomfortable if high light intensity is used.

Recording findings
Vitreous – floaters.
Neural retinal rim – pale nasal quadrant.
Disc margins – poorly defined.
Cup to disc ratio – value of ratio.
Crescents – choroidal.
Disc anomalies/abnormalities – tilting.
Vessels – tortuosity.
Fundus – pigmented.
Macula – haemorrhage.

Expected findings
Vitreous – clear.
Neural retinal rim – pink.
Disc margins – well defined.
Cup to disc ratio – (value of ratio).
Crescents – none, choroidal, scleral.
Disc anomalies/abnormalities – none.

Vessels – ¾ artery to vein ratio.
Fundus – healthy.
Macula – foveal reflex present.

Chapter 48 Diagnostic contact lens and gonioscopy

Introduction
This is a technique that allows accurate evaluation of the width anterior chamber angle and detailed inspection of the structures within the anterior segment of the eye. The angle is not normally visible using an ophthalmoscope or slit lamp, since light reflected by structures posterior to the limbus is totally internally reflected within the anterior chamber because of the curvature of the cornea. It is because of this phenomenon that sclerotic scatter illumination is possible. Also, the angle is concealed from direct observation by the projection of opaque scleral tissue over its anterior wall as far as the limbus. Gonioscopy is carried out using goniolenses of which there are several types. Most commonly used are the indirect mirrored lenses.

Indirect mirrored goniolenses are plastic cone-shaped contact lenses that are available in various sizes and designs containing one, two, three or four mirrors and a plano-concave lens in the centre of the cone apex, which effectively eliminates the cornea as a refracting surface. Any small difference in curvature between the lens and the cornea is minimized by interposing an optical coupling solution between the two surfaces, e.g. Viscotears lubricant.

The single-mirror goniolens is useful for teaching purposes and for those new to this technique, as the multi-mirrors of the three- and four-mirror versions can prove confusing for the novice. The single-mirror lens is considered a good choice for examining children, and adults with small palpebral apertures. In its three-mirror form the indirect goniolens (often known as the Goldmann 3-mirror) permits angle examination using the smallest arc-shaped internal mirror and a good view of the mid- and far-periphery of the fundus using the additional mirrors through a dilated pupil. As both the single- and three-mirror lenses only have one mirror positioned to view the angle, rotation through 360 degrees with an appropriate adjustment to the illumination is required. The slit lamp beam should always be approximately perpendicular to the base of the arc-shaped mirror. The Thorpe four-mirror and the Sussman four mirror goniolenses are designed to provide a view of the angle in each mirror. This is useful in that the lens has only to be rotated slightly in order for the complete angle to be observed. The Sussman four-mirror lens has an added advantage in that its small contact surface means that an optical coupling solution is not required to create an optical interface.

Use
Some optometrists are hesitant to dilate pupils for fear of precipitating an attack of closed angle glaucoma. Van Herick's slit lamp technique allows an approximation of

the openness of the angle, however the use of a goniolens will provide a more accurate evaluation of angle width as well as assessment of those structures discussed above, for anatomic anomalies and disease or the effects of trauma.

Slit lamp set up
- Coupled
- Beam straight ahead
- 2 mm beam width
- Maximum beam height
- No filter
- Medium illumination
- 10-15x magnification.

Procedure
As with all invasive procedures corneal health should be assessed using fluorescein in conjunction with the cobalt blue slit lamp filter.
The technique should not be carried out on a compromised cornea.
It is good practice before commencing gonioscopy to explain what is going to happen to the patient and why it is being done since the size of the lens can prove disconcerting.
The patient should be advised that the lens may feel strange but will not be uncomfortable.
This will usually reduce patient anxiety and improve co-operation.
The cornea should be anaesthetized with one drop of topical anaesthetic (e.g. Proxymetacaine 0.5%).
Bubble free coupling gel should be placed into the concavity of the goniolens.
With the patient looking up, the lower lid can be retracted with the fore-finger, then the lower lip of the lens inserted into the lower fornix, the upper lid is then lifted over the upper lip of the lens as the patient is instructed to look forward and the lens quickly pivoted onto the cornea with release of the upper lid.
The quicker this is done the less uncomfortable it is for the patient.
When using the single - and three-mirror lenses it is advisable to locate the arc-shaped mirror superiorly for orientation purposes.
In this position the inferior portion of the angle is available for inspection and as this is usually the widest part of the anterior chamber angle it enables the novice to more easily work out the relationship of the structures located there.
The left hand should be used to hold the lens when viewing the right eye.
The hand may be supported and held steady by the forehead strap or by resting the elbow on the slit lamp table.
For those with short arms a tissue box placed on the slit lamp table can provide added support.
By moving the slit lamp forward to focus on the reflected mirror image and by rotating the lens between forefinger and thumb gently through 360 degrees (less for the Thorpe and Sussman four-mirror goniolenses) the anterior chamber angle can be observed.
The goniolens can be removed by parting the lids so that they clear the lip of the lens. In most cases the lens will fall from the eye.

If the lens remains attached to the cornea by capillary attraction, the lateral sclera adjacent to the rim of the lens should be pressed firmly with the tip of one finger to break the capillary attraction holding the lens in place.

Hints and tips

The size of most goniolenses can make this procedure seem initially daunting for the patient and practitioner. It is in the interests of both that the practitioner learns how to insert the lens smoothly and quickly, even if the patient becomes anxious during the insertion stage.
Patient confidence in the practitioner will decrease if repeated attempts are required to insert the lens.
This often happens with a novice, as they are usually too pre-occupied with the patient's reaction as the lens is placed on the lower ready for insertion and not concentrating on the task at hand.
Once the lens is in place most beginners will mistake the optical artefact produced with in the cornea for features of interest. The cornea appears milky white due to internal reflection and is of little interest.
A brown thick line within this opaque region may be interpreted as the trabeculae meshwork or the ciliary body.
The novice should in fact approach the view from the other side of the angle and locate first the iris, then the last role of the iris and then the iris root.
Just above this will lie the structures of interest.
Deliberate compression (dynamic gonioscopy) gives the observer a certain amount of control over the iris configuration.
In an eye with a relatively narrow angle, deeper structures can be visualised by flattening the periphery of the iris gonioscopically.
It is also used to distinguish between true peripheral anterior synechiae and simple apposition of the iris to the cornea.
Note the type of mirrored lens that was used e.g. 3-mirror.

Recording findings

There are several types of notation system available that can be used to describe the openness of the anterior chamber angle.
They are all cumbersome to use in practice and it is acceptable to make a note of the most posterior structure visible in each quadrant of the angle.
Draw a large X where each compartment represents a quadrant of the angle.
The following abbreviations are suggested: CB ciliary body; SS scleral spur; TM trabecular meshwork; SL Schwalbe's line.

For example, RE

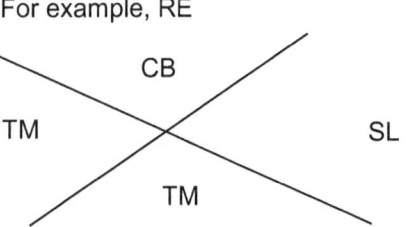

LE

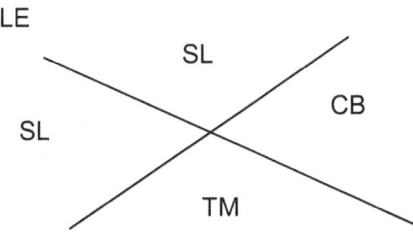

Chapter 49 Examination of the anterior chamber

Introduction
Examination of the anterior chamber is a technique that is important those eye care clinicians involved in the management of red eye. It is particularly useful in the differential diagnosis of glaucoma and iritis.

Van Herick anterior chamber depth estimation
The depth of the anterior chamber angle can be estimated by the van Herick technique. This is performed using a sharply focused optic section positioned on the cornea at the very edge of the limbus. The cornea will be seen in cross-section with the slit beam reflected off the front surface of the iris. In the presence of an open anterior chamber angle and clear aqueous humour, the anterior chamber is optically empty and appears as a black space between the cornea and iris. The width of the space formed by the anterior chamber angle relative to the width of the corneal section is used as a measure for the angle width estimation.

Use
This technique may elicit the first clinical sign of narrow-angle or acute angle closure glaucoma in the symptomatic patient who presents acutely. Angles that are identified as being very narrow with this technique should be further evaluated with a goniolens. Frequently angles will be shown to be larger with this procedure than the van Herick technique suggested. The technique can be used in the differential diagnosis of red eye e.g. viral conjunctivitis and closed angle glaucoma, closed angle and open angle glaucoma and acute and chronic glaucoma.

Slit lamp set up
- Coupled
- 60 degrees beam angle
- Beam width equivalent to an optic section
- Maximum beam height
- No filter
- Medium illumination
- 10-16X magnification.

Procedure
Place a narrow slit as close to the limbus as possible and normal to the cornea. Narrow the beam to an optic section and instruct the patient to look straight ahead. Focus the beam sharply on the cornea at the very edge of the temporal limbus. Compare the width of the 'shadow' formed on the iris (representing the depth of the anterior chamber) to the width of the optic section (representing the thickness of the cornea).

The shadow is a dark interval between the light on the cornea and the light on the iris, that represents the optically empty aqueous in the anterior chamber.
The procedure should be repeated for the nasal limbus.

The angle can be graded as follows:
- Grade 4-the ratio of aqueous to cornea is 1:1-open angle
- Grade 3-the ratio of aqueous to cornea is 1:2
- Grade 2-the ratio of aqueous to cornea is 1:4-indicates narrow angle, which should be viewed by gonioscopy
- Grade 1-the ratio is smaller than 1:4-indicates dangerously narrow angle, which is likely to close.

If the grades of the nasal and temporal angles are judged to be different, both readings should be recorded.

Hints and tips
Errors in angle estimation may occur if the patient's eyes are not in primary gaze. The most common mistake that will result in angle overestimation is if the optic section is not placed far enough peripherally at the corneoscleral junction.
The beam should be at exactly 60 degrees to the observation system.
Most slit lamps will have a scale for judging this angle.
Novice practitioners often have too wide a beam; it should be just thick enough to avoid extinction.

Recording findings
R van Herick angle nasal and temporal grade 3, L grade nasal grade 2 temporal grade 1.

Expected findings
R van Herick angle nasal and temporal grade ≥ 3, L van Herick angle nasal and temporal grade ≥ 3.

Smith anterior chamber depth estimation
This is another slit lamp procedure that can be used to estimate the depth of the anterior chamber. It provides a reliable means of anterior depth estimation and is simple and quick to perform. It may be carried out on any slit lamp that has a calibrated variable slit-length.

Slit lamp set up
- 60 degrees beam angle to the temporal side
- Maximum slit length
- Moderate illumination
- Magnification x10
- The right eyepiece is used for the right eye and vice versa.

Use
This technique may elicit the first clinical sign of narrow-angle or acute angle closure glaucoma in the symptomatic patient who presents acutely. Angles that are identified

as being very narrow with this technique should be further evaluated with a goniolens. The technique can be used in the differential diagnosis of red eye e.g. viral conjunctivitis and closed angle glaucoma, closed angle and open angle glaucoma and acute and chronic glaucoma.

Procedure
With the patient looking straight ahead a 1 to 2 mm wide slit beam is orientated horizontally and is focused on the cornea.
A second image of the slit is formed by the anterior lens capsule/iris.
Beginning with a short beam, the beam width is slowly increased.
This reduces the gap between the corneal and lenticular/iris slits.
The length of the beam is further increased until the two appear to be just touching.
The beam length that yields this is the end point.
The slit length at the end point is multiplied by a correction factor of 1.31 to obtain the anterior chamber angle depth in mm.

Hints and tips
Always set the illumination system at 60 degrees compared to the observation system.
Don't make the beam too narrow - approximately 3mm is ideal.
Always use the right eye to view the patient's right eye as this is a monocular technique, or the results will be variable and the same for the left eye.

Recording findings
Smith's technique anterior chamber depth R 2.5, L 3 mm.

Expected findings
Smith's technique anterior chamber depth R and L 3 to 4 mm.

Anterior chamber evaluation using the Tyndall effect
Introduction
The aqueous humour is normally virtually optically empty so that the anterior chamber appears black when the slit beam passes through it. In the presence of anterior uveitis, protein and white blood cells leak into the anterior chamber from inflamed blood vessels of the iris and ciliary body. The Tyndall effect will allow the visualisation of these small particles as they circulate in the anterior chamber via the aqueous convection currents.

Use
This technique is particularly useful for evaluating the anterior chamber for cells and flare due to anterior uveitis. White blood cells appear as whitish specks while protein is not visible as discrete particles but gives an overall milky appearance to the aqueous. The grading of cells and flare is determined by the quantity of each visible at any one time in the slit lamp beam. A grade of 0 (none or trace) to 4 (severe) is given to both. Pigment particles from the iris pigment epithelium may be released into the anterior chamber angle following blunt trauma, routine pupillary dilation, and in patients with pigment dispersion syndrome. Assessing the status of the anterior chamber is essential to the accurate differential diagnosis of acute ocular infections

and inflammations, especially following traumatic insult. In a non-inflamed eye, keratic precipitates on the corneal endothelium may suggest chronic uveitis.

Slit lamp set up
- Coupled
- 60 degrees beam angle positioned temporally
- Conic section or parallelepiped 1 mm wide and 2 mm high
- No filter
- Maximum illumination with room lights off
- 25-40x magnification.

Procedure
Performing oscillatory movements of a conic section or parallelepiped, focused on the central cornea and then on the anterior surface of the lens for 30 to 60 seconds, will highlight the presence of anterior chamber cells and flare (protein)
Due to the minute size of this debris, maximum illumination and magnification obtainable with the biomicroscope are required to evaluate the anterior chamber.

Hints and tips
A room with reduced or extinguished lighting is required.
It is necessary to wait for at least 30 seconds in order to dark-adapt before carrying out this procedure. A small intense slit should be used.
The novice clinician will usually overlook mild to moderate anterior uveitis because of the subtleness of the findings.
It is very important to use the maximum illumination and magnification settings of the slit lamp and to dark-adapt.
Following the initial evaluation pupillary dilation to increase the amount of black pupillary background area will facilitate visualization of the cells and flare.

Recording findings
Anterior chamber R cells grade 2, no flare, L cells grade 0, flare grade 4.

Expected findings
R and L anterior chamber optically empty.

Chapter 50 Examination of the iris

Introduction
Examination of the anterior chamber is a technique that is important for those eye care clinicians involved in the management of red eye and the monitoring of patients with glaucoma. It is particularly useful in the differential diagnosis of iritis, where the pupil margin may be irregular and pigment dispersion syndrome where the iris is likely to transilluminate.

Use
The iris can be examined for signs that may suggest current or previous glaucomatous disease. Iris transillumination can be carried out simply and quickly by retro-illuminating the iris with light reflected from the retina in a darkened room depigmented areas of the iris may be visible. Anterior and posterior synechiae can be detected using direct illumination of the iris and rear surface of the cornea and the iris and anterior surface of the crystalline lens, respectively.

Slit lamp set up
- Coupled
- Use a wide parallelepiped
- Set the illumination arm 30 to 45 degrees from the straight-ahead position
- Use a medium magnification setting 6-10X.

Procedure
Scan across the iris surface, looking for irregularities.
Note the pupillary light reflex.
The pupil should constrict when the slit lamp beam reaches the pupillary margin.

Hints and tips
Start with the beam totally extinguished and then slowly open up the beam width adjustor until a thin beam appears.
Continue opening up the adjustor until the beam width is approximately 2mm. The beam will now have the shape of a parallelepiped.

Recording findings
R iris transillumination and irregular pupil margin, L posterior synechiae 2 to 6 o'clock.

Expected findings
R and L no transillumination, iris quiet.

Chapter 51 Examination of the vitreous

Introduction
The focal length of the slit lamp allows for observation of approximately the anterior one third of the vitreous body. Use of auxiliary instrumentation such as multi-mirrored lenses and positive condensing lenses will extend the focal range of the slit lamp further into the posterior chamber for more extensive examination of the vitreous. Vitreous evaluation is best performed following pupillary dilation and the most useful illumination technique is direct focal illumination. The parallelepiped and optic section procedures can be used for vitreous evaluation. The former produces a three dimensional section of the vitreous and is most useful.

Direct focal illumination
This refers to the focusing of the light beam and the microscope in the same area. It does not refer to the coaxial placement of the light source with the microscope. The parallelepiped and optical section are two commonly used types of direct illumination. The parallelepiped illuminates a three-dimensional tissue area and is effective for detecting tissue lesions. An optic section illuminates a two dimensional area of tissue that is viewed obliquely and is used to localise the depth of lesions. It is used to examine the cornea and in particular to determine the depth of any compromise.

Use
The anterior portion of the vitreous appears as milky folds of gossamer-like texture separated by optically empty spaces. These folds appear wavy and oscillate with eye movements. In the very young patient the collagen fibrils are difficult to distinguish. In the older patient, however, the folds are seen to be composed of individual crisscrossing fibrils.

Indications for slit lamp examination of the vitreous include symptoms of floaters and light flashes, to diagnose posterior vitreous detachment with or without retinal complication, and to assess vitreous involvement in intraocular segment inflammation. Several conditions may result in inflammatory cells, red blood cells, or pigment cells moving into the vitreous. These cells will appear as small punctate opacities, suspended or slowly floating within the optically empty spaces between the fibrils and in the retrolental space. Red-brown vitreous cells are very likely to be red blood cells and/or retinal pigment epithelial (RPE) cells. Known as tobacco dusting or Shaffer's sign, these red-brown cells are usually an indication that a retinal tear or detachment is present so that the RPE cells have become dislodged or associated retinal vessel damage has occurred.

Slit lamp set up for a parallelepiped
- Coupled
- 60 degrees beam angle
- 1-2 mm beam width
- Maximum beam height
- No filter
- Medium illumination
- 10-16X magnification
- Use the joystick to sharply focus the microscope and the parallelepiped simultaneously.

Slit lamp set up for an optic section
- Coupled
- 60 degrees beam angle
- Beam width nearly extinguished
- Maximum beam height
- No filter
- Medium illumination
- 10-16X magnification
- Use the joystick to sharply focus the microscope and the optic section simultaneously.

Procedure
Starting at the temporal border of the dilated right pupil, move the joystick forward to focus the parallelepiped into the anterior vitreous.
Keep this portion of the vitreous in focus while scanning across to the nasal pupil.
Move the joystick further forward so as to focus into the vitreous as far as possible and scan across it to the temporal pupil border.
Repeating this with the beam positioned nasally will allow thorough examination

Hints and tips
Significant cataract formation can obscure the various vitreous landmarks.
A good deal of observation skill development is needed to accurately assess the presence of vitreous cells.
Also the collapse of the posterior limiting layer of the vitreous in posterior vitreous detachment (PVD) can be easily over looked if the slit lamp is not focussed well into the posterior chamber.
Instruct the patient to move the eye around in order to stir up any vitreal debris.
To distinguish between red blood cells and pigment particles introduce the red free (green) filter.
Red blood cells will appear black and will no longer be visible within the vitreous.
Pigment particles will not absorb the red-free light and will still be visible.

Recording findings
R vitreous pigment particles, L vitreous red blood cells.

Expected findings
R and L vitreous optically empty.

SECTION 6 SPECIALIST BINOCULAR VISION

Chapter 52 Monocular estimate method (MEM) dynamic retinoscopy

Chapter 53 Low neutral dynamic retinoscopy

Chapter 54 Accommodative facility

Chapter 55 Vergence facility

Chapter 56 Detection of ARC using the Mallett Unit

Chapter 57 Bagolini lenses

Chapter 58 Determination of AC/A ratio

Chapter 59 Eccentric fixation

Chapter 60 Jump convergence

Chapter 61 Prism cover test

Chapter 62 Fusional reserves

Chapter 52 Monocular estimate method (MEM) dynamic retinoscopy

Introduction
In the monocular estimate method (MEM) of dynamic retinoscopy the amount of the lag of accommodation is estimated by judging the width, speed and brightness of the retinoscopic reflex.

Procedure
The test card and the retinoscope should be placed at the same distance from the subject's spectacle plane, usually 40 cm.
With the retinoscope in the plane mirror mode, with motion indicates a lag of accommodation and an against motion indicates a lead of accommodation while neutrality indicates that the accommodative stimulus and accommodative response are equal.
The practitioner's estimate of the amount of plus power that would be required to neutralise the with motion is the estimate of the lag of accommodation.
The estimate of the lag can be confirmed by very briefly placing a plus lens equal in power to the estimated lag over one eye and quickly checking to see whether neutrality is observed.
The lens should only be in place a half-second or less so that a change in accommodative response is not induced.
Record the dioptric power of the lens that provides neutrality
Repeat procedure for the L eye.

Hints and tips
Plus lenses indicate positive accommodative lag (response < stimulus).
Minus lenses indicate negative accommodative lag (response > stimulus).
Lag > +1.00DS indicates accommodative insufficiency.
Lag < 0 indicates latent hyperopia, pseudomyopia or accommodative spasm.
School age children are reported to have a mean lag of 0.34D.
Most non-presbyopic subjects have lags of 0 to 0.75D with MEM retinoscopy.

Recording findings
MEM RE +1.000DS LE +1.00DS.

Expected findings
R and L zero to +0.75DS.

Chapter 53 Low neutral dynamic retinoscopy

Introduction
Low neutral dynamic retinoscopy yields the lens power with which the dioptric accommodative stimulus and dioptric accommodative response are equal.

Procedure
The retinoscope and the test card are maintained at the same distance from the subject, usually 40 cm from the spectacle plane.
Testing is started with the subject's distance refractive correction in place.
If a lag is observed, plus lenses are added in 0.25D steps until a neutral retinoscopic reflex is observed.
The lens power added for neutrality is recorded. If, for example, the test result is +0.75D with a 40 cm distance, then the accommodative stimulus is 0.75D less than the 2.50D for the test distance, or 1.75D. Since the neutral was observed at that point, the accommodative response is also 1.75D.
If an 'against' movement is seen with the retinoscope and 'budgie stick' at 40 cm i.e. a lag < 0, latent hyperopia, pseudomyopia or accommodative spasm is indicated.
If a 'with' movement is seen with the text and retinoscope at 40 cm and no movement is seen when the retinoscope moved out to 67 cm but the text remains at 40 cm then 2.50 (40 cm) – 1.50 (67 cm) = lag of +1.00DS.

Recording findings
Low neutral dynamic ret. R +1.25D, L+1.50D.

Expected findings
If reflex is 'with' the retinoscope at 67 cm and the text at 40 cm then lag would be expected to be between zero and +1.00D.

Chapter 54 Accommodative facility

Introduction
Accommodative facility is a measure of the speed of accommodative change. The dioptric accommodative stimulus is alternated between two different levels and the subject reports when a letter target is seen clearly after each alternation in accommodative stimulus. The examiner counts the number of cycles completed in one minute (one cycle being the change from one stimulus level to the other and back again). Accommodative stimulus can be varied either by lens power changes or by viewing distance changes. The first is referred to as 'lens rock' and the second as 'distance rock', indicating that the accommodative stimulus is 'rocked' back and forth. The standard method of testing accommodative facility is a lens rock procedure using a pair of +2.00D lenses on one side of a flipper bar and -2.00D lenses on the other side.

Use
This test is useful in those cases when the patient has visual symptoms which such a problem with accommodation but the amplitudes of accommodation are measured as being in the normal range.

Procedure
Room lights on.
Patient wears distance correction (if appropriate).
Explain to patient: I am going to test your ability to change focus.
The test starts with the +2.00D lenses over the subject's refractive correction.
A test distance of 40 cm is usually used with the reduced Snellen letters at a 6/6 to 6/12 VA demand.
This type of target has no suppression control and for children younger than six years of age, it is more appropriate to use the OXO target on the near Mallett unit. With the polarising filters in place the vertical fixation disparity bars can be used to check for suppression.
Occlude LE.
Explain: Keep looking at the word. I will place a lens in front of your eye that may make the word appear blurred. I want you to focus and make the print clear again. As soon as it becomes clear, say 'clear'. I will then flip another lens in front of your eye that may make the word blurry again. As before, I want you to focus and make the work clear again, and then say 'clear'. I will repeat this for 30 seconds.
Use a watch to time 60 seconds.
Hold the +2.00DS flipper lens in place until patient says 'clear'.
Quickly flip the -2.00DS lens in place until the patient says 'clear'.
Count the number of times that the plus and minus lenses (representing 1 cycle) are 'cleared' in 60 seconds.

Occlude RE, and repeat 1 to 10 for LE.
Repeat above procedure with both eyes open.

Hints and tips
During binocular 'lens rock' testing, adjustments in fusional vergence must occur to compensate for the changes in accommodative vergence. Therefore, subjects may pass the monocular lens rock but fail the binocular lens rock facility if a vergence disorder is present.

Some clinicians suggest that it may be more appropriate to train the monocular accommodative facility prior to the binocular facility, especially if the binocular lens rock performance is limited by fusional vergence dysfunction. In this case it would be appropriate to use reduced Snellen letters, since suppression would not be a problem.

Recording findings
Record as number of cycles per minute, e.g. accommodative facility (±2.00DS) RE 11cpm, LE 11cpm, BE 8cpm.

Expected findings
Cut-offs for test failure used by many clinicians using +2.00D/-2.00D flippers and a 40 cm viewing distance for children and adults up to 30 years of age are less than 11 cycles per minute for monocular testing and less than 8 cycles per minute for binocular testing.
Some suggest that these criteria should be dropped to 5cpm (monocular) and 2.5cpm (binocular) in children of 8-12 years.

Chapter 55 Vergence facility

Introduction
Vergence facility can be assessed with prism flippers. It is defined as the number of cycles per minute (cpm) that a stimulus can be fused through alternating base-in and base out prism, and attempts to capture the ability of the fusional vergence system to respond rapidly and accurately to changing vergence demands over time. Various combinations of base-in and base-out lenses have been have been described in the literature, including 4Δ base-in/16Δ base-out, 5Δ base-in/15Δ base-out and 8Δ base-in/8Δ base-out. Most texts and research papers describing this procedure suggest the use of 8Δ base-in/8Δ base-out flippers.

Use
Vergence facility is a measure of stamina and sustaining ability of the vergence system. He former is assessed by turning the flipper so that the patient looks at a near target through the base-in and then the base-out. The latter refers to the ability to maintain vergence at a particular level, rather than to rapidly alter the level, for a sustained period of time and can be assessed by holding the prism flipper in front of the eyes until the patient experiences ocular discomfort. The test is useful for those patients complaining of near vision symptoms that suggest a vergence problem but the near point of convergence is in the normal range. This test is carried out with both the patient's eyes open usually involves measurement of stamina rather than sustainability.

Procedure
Room lights on.
Patient should wear an appropriate refractive correction allowing for any presbyopia and the near testing distance
Explain: I am going to test your ability to change eye focus.
A test distance of 40 cm is usually used with the reduced Snellen letters at a 6/6 to 6/12 acuity demand.
This type of target has no suppression control and for children younger than six years of age, it is more appropriate to use the OXO target on the near Mallett unit
With the polarising filters in place the vertical fixation disparity bars can be used to check for suppression.
Explain: Keep looking at the letters. I will place a lens in front of your eye that may make the word appear blurred and double. I want you to focus and make the print clear and single. As soon as it becomes clear and single, say 'clear and single'. I will then flip another lens in front of your eye that may make the letters blurry and double again. As before, I want you to focus and make the work clear and single again, and then say 'clear and single'. I will repeat this for 60 seconds.
Use a watch to time 60 seconds.

The test starts with the 8Δ prism base-out over the subject's refractive correction, wait until the patient says 'clear and single'.
Quickly flip the 8Δ base-in prism in place until the patient says 'clear and single'
Count the number of times that the plus and minus lenses (representing 1 cycle) are 'cleared and made single' in 60 seconds.

Hints and tips
A few practice flips may be necessary to allow the patient to become familiar with the test.
Encourage the patient during the test as they might find it slightly uncomfortable when trying to overcome the base-in prism.
Use only the cpm value to aid in clinical decision making and ignore any subjective difficulty or comments from the patient.

Recording findings
Record as number of cycles per minute (cpm) along with the prism combination used, e.g. vergence facility (8Δ base-in/8Δ base-out) 15 cpm.

Expected findings
With 4Δ base-in/16Δ base-out flippers one study showed that 5 year olds had a mean of 7.6 cpm and 12 year olds had a mean of 13.0 cpm. With a 5Δ base-in/15Δ base-out and 8Δ base-in/8Δ base-out flippers mean values were similar for the two tests, ranging from 11.3 to 14.1 cpm. Others have used 3Δ base-in/12Δ base-out combinations and found an 'expected' value of 13.41 ± 3.68 cpm. Using this prism combination anything less than 15 cpm was considered to be clinically significant and anything less than 12 cpm 'should reliably detect symptomatic children'.

Chapter 56 Detection of ARC using the Mallett Unit

Introduction
As well as being used to detect fixation disparity the Mallett Unit can be used to detect global and local suppression in the presence of small to medium angle comitant strabismus.

Use
The instrument is particular useful in assisting with differential diagnosis when patients present with a slight to moderate unilateral reduction in visual acuity that does not improve with a pinhole. Some patients with this type of presentation will have a small angle strabismus that is not detectable using the cover test (microtropia with identity). Proving the existence of ARC in this type of case will help rule out more sinister causes for the unilateral reduction in visual acuity. The presence of ARC is also important in determining the prognosis for obtaining binocular function in patients with a heterotropia. It is not a routine test and only needs to be carried out when investigating the level of binocularity of patients with a heterotropia.

Procedure
Ask the patient to hold the near Mallett Unit at their usual near working distance. This distance may be exactly measured using the retractable tape measure incorporated in the housing of the unit.
The refractive error including any presbyopic addition has to be in the trial frame. Direct the patient to look at the X of the small OXO (with vertical green markers) and to be aware but not directly look at the green markers.
Without the polarizing visor in place the markers should be centrally aligned with the X and two will be present.
This gives the patient a reference point of how the markers should be positioned and how many there should be.

Place the polarizing visor in the trial frame and ask if two green markers are still visible one above and one below the X.
If only one line is seen then there is central suppression in the eye that should see the missing marker.
The patient should now be directed to the larger OXO in the top left hand corner of the Mallett unit (only more recent versions have this) and if both green lines can be seen with the polarizing visor in place then in the presence of a small angle comitant strabismus the presence of ARC has been indirectly proved.

Hints and tips
The smaller green line falls in the central suppression scotoma and is therefore not seen.
The larger green line is much larger than the central suppression scotoma classically associated with ARC and is therefore seen.
Some patients may comment that the green lines above and below the large OXO are visible but one is displaced slightly to the side of the centre (the marker that is seen by the deviated eye).
This is not indicative of a fixation disparity type of slip but relates to the eye misalignment (the exact mechanism is unknown) and this displacement should be ignored.
Some versions of the near Mallett Unit do not have the large OXO target.
The distance unit can be used in a similar way to that described for the near unit but the working distance has to be 1.5 m in order for the red markers to subtend an appropriate angle of arc.
The larger the heterotropia the less likely that ARC will be detected with this (or any other) technique.
ARC does not need to be treated, as the visual acuity is likely to be at least 6/12 and the cosmesis good.
While the Mallett unit can be used to prove the presence of ARC no information on the depth of ARC is obtained.

Recording findings
Mallett Unit, ARC detected RE.

Chapter 57 Bagolini lenses

Introduction
Bagolini lenses are available in a reversible lorgnette or trial lens form. Each plane glass lens has fine parallel striations inscribed onto the surface orientated at 45 degrees on one lens and 135 degrees on the other. A spotlight is converted into a line image seen at 90 degrees to the striations when viewed through the lenses. Bagolini lenses test ARC under the most natural conditions (minimally dissociative) when compared to other tests for ARC.

Use
The test is particular useful in assisting with differential diagnosis when patients present with a slight to moderate unilateral reduction in visual acuity that does not improve with a pinhole. Some patients with this type of presentation will have a small angle strabismus that is not detectable using the cover test (microtropia with identity). Proving the existence of ARC in this type of case will help rule out more sinister causes for the unilateral reduction in visual acuity. The presence of ARC is also important in determining the prognosis for obtaining binocular function in patients with a heterotropia. It is not a routine test and only needs to be carried out when investigating the level of binocularity of patients with a heterotropia.

Procedure
Unilateral heterotropia
Room lights on.
With any refractive correction *in situ* ask the patient to fixate a spotlight at 6m. Place a Bagolini lens in front of the deviating eye, with the striations positioned at 180°. Carry out the test with both eyes open and explain: This test examines how your eyes work together.
Have a pencil and paper ready for the patient to describe/draw what they see.
Ask: Please look at the spotlight and draw what you can see.
May need to ask:
How many spotlights can you see? (Diplopia?)
Can you see a line? (Suppression?)
Does line have a gap? (Foveal suppression scotoma?)

Possible results:
- A line centred on the spotlight means the presence of binocular single vision or harmonious ARC.
- Differentiation can be made using the cover test, which would normally elicit a small heterotropia if ARC were present.
- A gap in one of the lines indicates the presence of a foveal suppression scotoma (rarely reported by patients in our experience).

Art of Clinical Practice in Optometry

- A displaced line and spot indicates the presence of a heterotropia with NRC.
- Confirmation can be made by adding prism strength equal to the angle of deviation.
- A dot with a line going through the middle will be produced in NRC but crossed projection will occur in an esotropic patient with ARC.
- One spotlight but no line image means central and peripheral suppression.
- See Figure 37 for examples of recording findings.

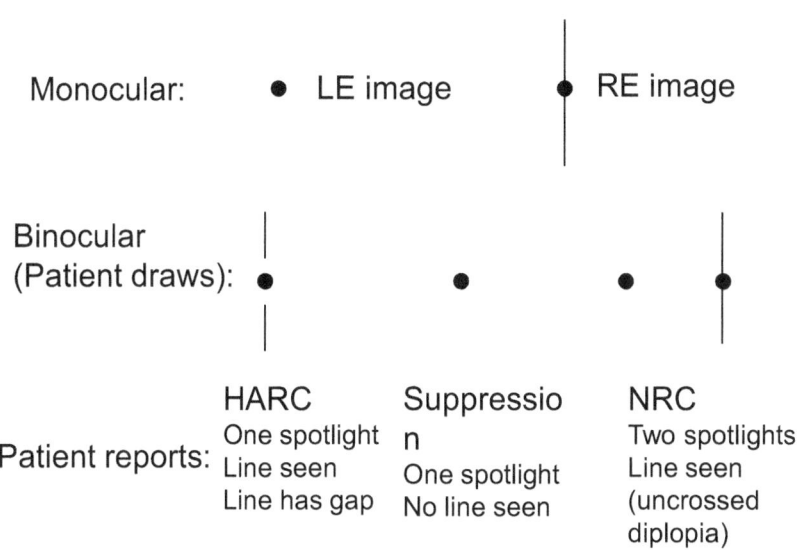

Figure 37 Recording findings with a single Bagolini lens: right esotropia.

Procedure
Alternating heterotropia
Room lights on.
With any refractive correction *in situ* ask the patient to fixate a spotlight at 6m. Place Bagolini lenses in front of both eyes, striations at 45 & 135°. Carry out test with both eyes open and explain: This test examines how your eyes work together.
Have a pencil and paper ready for the patient to draw what they see.
Ask: Please look at the spotlight and describe/draw what you can see.
May need to ask:
How many spotlights can you see? (Diplopia?)
Can you see a line? (Suppression?)
Does the line have a gap?' (Foveal suppression scotoma?)
Displaced lines indicate heterotropia with NRC.
Confirmation can be made by adding prism strength equal to the angle of deviation.

A dot with a line going through the middle will be produced in NRC but crossed projection will occur in an esotropic patient with ARC.

One spotlight with one line means central and peripheral suppression. See Figure 38 for examples of recording findings.

Hints and tips

Use one only Bagolini lens if the heterotropia is unilateral and constant as this will keep dissociation to a minimum.

Always use a Bagolini lens in front of each eye if the heterotropia is of the alternating type.

Look behind the Bagolini lenses to check which eye is fixing when asking the patient to describe/draw the images.

If the patient does not report a gap in the line image that corresponds to the deviating eye but all the other clinical signs suggest the presence of a small angle deviation and ARC then it is very likely that the gap is too small for the patient to detect.

The larger the heterotropia the less likely that ARC will be detected with this (or any other) technique.

ARC does not need to be treated, as the visual acuity is likely to be at least 6/12 and the cosmesis good.

While Bagolini lenses can be used to prove the presence of ARC no information on the depth of ARC is obtained.

The larger the heterotropia the less likely that ARC will be detected with this (or any other) technique.

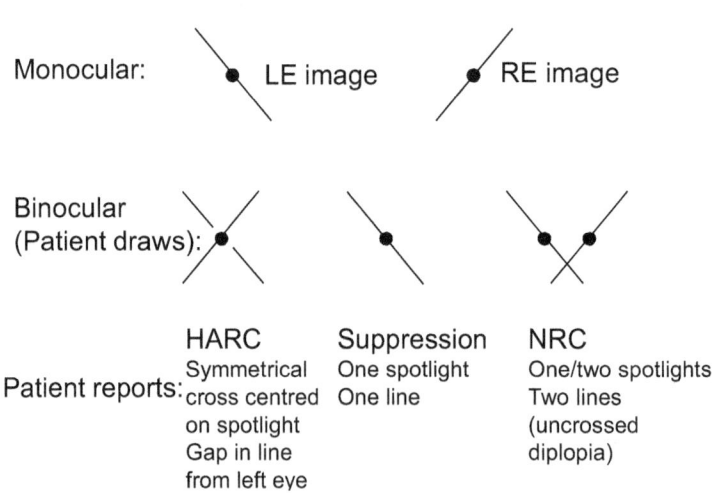

Figure 38 Recording findings with a single Bagolini lens: alternating esotropia right eye fixation.

Chapter 58 Determination of the AC/A ratio

Introduction
The AC/A ratio determines the amount of accommodative convergence induced in response to one dioptre of accommodation. The normal ratio is between 2 to 4:1 i.e. 2 to 4 dioptres of convergence are produced from each dioptre of accommodation. Unless there is surgical intervention the ratio is maintained until the onset of presbyopia. If the ratio is higher or lower than normal, over or under convergence may produce a heterotropia.

Use
The size of the ratio is important in certain cases regarding whether management should take a conservative or surgical course. Measurement is indicated in:

- All cases in which there is a significant difference between the size of the distance and near deviations
- Intermittent esotropia of the convergence excess type
- Intermittent distance exotropia to differentiate between true and simulated types

Determination of the AC/A ratio is useful for some pre-presbyopes and particularly for children with near eso- or exotropia. Measurement after 45 years of age is of little value.

Procedure
The gradient and calculated methods will be described here. The gradient method can be used with concave lenses at 6m for convergence excess deviations or convex lenses at 33cm for divergence excess deviations.

Using concave lenses
With any refractive correction *in situ* in a trial frame, the deviation is measured using the prism cover test at 6m (or Maddox rod) using a detailed fixation target
With -3.00DS lenses in a trail frame the distance prism cover test (or Maddox rod) should be repeated using the same target provided it can still be seen clearly
If sufficient exertion of accommodation is not possible the ratio should be calculated using either –2.00DS or –1.00DS.

Calculation of ratio
PCT = Prism cover test
MR = Maddox rod
MW = Maddox wing

AC/A = PCT (or MR) value in the active state – PCT (or MR) value in the non-active state/strength of the lens used.

For example, in convergence excess esotropia:

PCT (or MR) with –3.00DS = 25Δ base-out
PCT (or MR) without –3.00DS = 4Δ base-out
AC/A ratio = $\frac{+25 - (+4)}{3}$ = 7:1Δ/D i.e. a high ratio

Using convex lenses
The method is the same as for concave lenses but the fixation target should be at 33cm and convex lenses used.
If the patient cannot relax the accommodation by 3 DS then +2.00DS or +1.00DS can be used.

For example, in a distance exotropia:

PCT (or MW) without +3.00DS = 10Δ base-in
PCT (or MW) with +3.00DS = 35Δ base-in

AC/A ratio = $\frac{-10 - (-35)}{3}$ = 8:1Δ/D i.e. a high ratio

Calculated AC/A method
Procedure
Take distance (measured with a prism bar or the Maddox Rod) and near (measured with a prism bar or the Maddox Wing) heterophoria and apply to the following formula:

AC/A = PD + [(n − d) ÷ D]

where: PD = interpupillary distance e.g. 6cm
n = near phoria e.g. −4Δ (XOP)
d = distance phoria e.g. 0 Δ (ortho)
D = accommodation i.e. 3.33D.

AC/A = 6 + {(-4 - 0) ÷ 3.33} = 4.8Δ/D
This method does not control proximal accommodation and convergence as it is carried out at two distances

Recording findings
Record method, calculated/modified gradient test and the value.

Expected findings
AC/A (calculated) 4Δ/D.

Chapter 59 Eccentric fixation

Introduction
Eccentric fixation (EF) exists only in amblyopic eyes. It is common in strabismic amblyopia and rare in anisometropic amblyopia. It occurs when the amblyopic eye attempts to fixate with an off-foveal point under monocular conditions. Visual acuity is affected so it is important to be aware of it clinically. Eccentric fixation with a non-foveal point leads to a linear decrease in visual acuity the further fixation is from the fovea. Most esotropic patients exhibit nasal EF and those who are exotropic exhibit temporal EF. The cause of EF is unknown.

Visuoscopy is the procedure used to assess EF. It is the same as direct ophthalmoscopy but a grid target on an ophthalmoscope is used to determine the presence of eccentric fixation, as well as its magnitude and direction. This procedure can be performed successfully on an undilated pupil. Visuoscopy *must* be done with the patient's eye not being tested occluded because eccentric fixation is a monocular condition.

In order to perform visuoscopy, focus the grid target of the ophthalmoscope on the retina of the amblyopic eye while asking the patient to view the centre of the 'bull's eye' target.

Central fixation reveals the foveal reflex directly in the centre of the grid. Eccentric fixation is represented by the foveal reflex located outside the centre of the grid.

The examiner must identify the retinal location the patient is using to fixate.

Procedure
Use a Visuscope on suspect eye as when conducting direct ophthalmoscopy.
Focus the grid on the macula.
Cover over patient's good eye with your or their hand.
Ask patient to look at centre of grid.
Compare position of foveal reflex with centre of grid.
Foveal reflex gives position of actual fovea.
If the foveal reflex does not coincide with centre of target person has EF.

Note the magnitude and direction of eccentricity; each mark on the grid represents 1 prism dioptre of EF, the direction of EF is represented by where the grid lies in respect to the foveal reflex. See Figure 39.

Steadiness must be noted-most amblyopic patients demonstrate unsteady fixation.

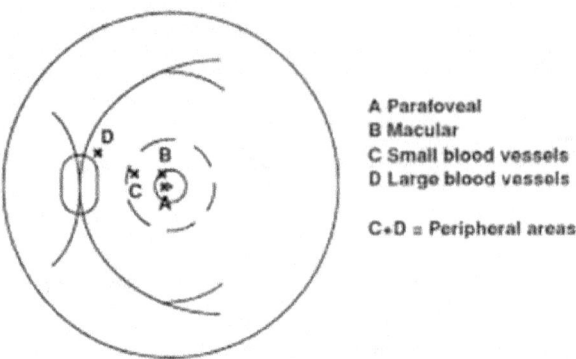

Figure 39 Magnitude and direction of eccentric fixation

Chapter 60 Jump convergence

Introduction
Jump convergence is the ability to alternate convergence between two targets, one distant and one near.

Use
This test provides further information about the vergence system and is especially useful for those patients that have with symptoms associated with near work.

Procedure
Room lights on.
Appropriate near refractive correction worn.
Illuminate near target with local light if necessary.
Explain: This test determines how well your eyes change convergence between distant and near objects.
Point to a letter on the distance chart (one line above VA of patient's poorer eye) and explain: This is the distant target.
Hold a pen tip at 15 cm from patient and explain: This is the near target.
Instruct: Please keep looking from the distant object to the near object and back again until I say stop.
Observe the quality of convergence and divergence and check that binocular fixation is maintained.

Recording findings
If movements are smooth and fast then record: Jump good to 15 cm.
If movements are jerky then record: Jump: poor to 15 cm.

Hints and tips
Compared to a remote NPC, poor jump convergence may be:
More prevalent
More closely associated with symptoms.
Jump convergence is not routinely measured but should be considered if:
Symptoms are suggestive of convergence insufficiency even if NPC is normal.

Chapter 61 Prism cover test

Introduction
The prism cover test is an objective dissociative method of measuring the total angle of deviation using horizontal and/or vertical prisms. Torsional deviations cannot be measured using this technique.
Angles of deviation should be measured at 6 m and 33 cm in the primary position of gaze.
The test may also be used to measure deviations at different distances or fields of gaze, depending upon findings from the history, cover test and oculomotility assessment.
Results from the cover test and oculomotility assessment will provide information on the approximate size and components of the deviation, the preferred eye for fixation and whether the deviation is concomitant or incomitant.

Equipment required
Horizontal and vertical prism bars and loose square prisms.
Detailed fixation targets, selected appropriately for the age of the patient and level of visual acuity of each eye.
Occluder (for younger patients, the palm of the examiner's hand may be more suitable).

Procedure
The patient is required to fixate a target at 6 m. A prism strength approximating the size of the deviation should then be placed in front of the deviating eye in heterotropia, with the apex in the direction of the deviation, or either eye in heterophoria.
An alternate cover test should be performed, gradually increasing the prism strength until the movement of the eye is reversed. The size of the deviation is recorded as the prism value just before reversal.
The procedure should be routinely repeated for 33 cm, and, when indicated, in other fields of gaze (maintain the fixation target in the primary position while the patient's head is moved to place the eyes in the required position), fixation distances, and when fixing with each eye in the case of incomitancy

It is essential to:
> Prevent fusion and elicit the total deviation-for maximum dissociation allow sufficient time (at least two seconds) for the patient to fixate the target accurately, followed by a quick movement of the occluder to the other eye
> Maintain and control accommodation by using a detailed fixation target appropriate for the patient's age.

Simultaneous prism cover test
Introduction
This is a modification of the prism cover test and is used to measure the heterotropic component of a deviation that has heterotropic and heterophoric components, for instance in some cases of microtropia. Assessment of the size of the heterotropia enables more accurate classification of the type of deviation.

Procedure
The prism is placed in front of the deviating eye and a cover-uncover test is performed only on the fixing eye.
Prism and cover are removed and the test is repeated with larger prisms.
The deviation is therefore measured using minimum dissociation until the point of reversal. The size of the manifest component is recorded as the prism value just before reversal of the eye movement.

Recording findings
25 alt XOT with 4 RhyperT-alternating tropia (prism bar used).

Expected findings
This depends on the size of any heterotropia and heterophoria present.

Chapter 62 Fusional reserves

Introduction
Fusional reserves are the amount of fusional vergence that can be exerted to maintain clear and single binocular vision. Components of fusional vergence are:

Sensory fusion - the ability to appreciate two similar images, one formed on each retina and interpret them as a single image.
Motor fusion - the maintenance of sensory fusion during vergence movements.

Procedure
Room lights on.
Appropriate near refractive correction worn.
Illuminate near target with local light if necessary.
Explain: This test measures the range over which your eye muscles can keep objects single.
Point to letter on distance chart (line above VA of poorer eye) and explain: Please look at this letter on the chart.
Use prism bar.

Distance negative fusional reserves (NFR of base-in vergences)
Use base-in prisms.
RE diverges (negative fusional vergence) due to fusion reflex.
Hold prism bar (zero prism) over RE.
Instruct: Please tell me when the letter goes double.
Slowly increase base-in prism, encourage patient to maintain single vision when diplopia first reported.
Make mental note of prism value that gives rise to sustained diplopia = break point.
Instruct: Please tell me when the letter goes single again.
Slowly reduce base-in prism until single vision is restored and make a mental note of prism value = recovery point.

Distance positive fusional reserves (PFR of base-out vergences)
Use base-out prisms.
RE converges (positive fusional vergence) due to fusion reflex.
Hold prism bar (zero prism) over RE.
Instruct: Please tell me when the letter goes blurred.
Slowly increase base-out prism; encourage patient to maintain clear vision when first blurs; mental note of prism value that gives sustained blur = blur point.
Measure break point and recovery point as for NFR.

Distance vertical fusional reserves
Right infra-vergence (R infra or base-up/RE).
RE depresses due to fusion reflex.
Increase bas-up prism more slowly than for horizontal fusional reserves (FR).
Measure break point and recovery point.
Right supravergence (R supra or base-down/RE).
RE depresses due to fusion reflex.
Increase BD prism more slowly than for horizontal FR.
Measure break point and recovery point.

Near fusional reserves
Room lights on.
Appropriate near refractive correction worn.
Point to letter on near chart (line above VA of poorer eye) at appropriate distance and explain: Please look at this letter on the chart.
Illuminate target with local light if necessary.
Use prism bar to measure:
NFR: blur / break / recovery
PFR: blur / break / recovery
R infra: break / recovery
R supra: break / recovery.

Recording findings
Record: blur/break/recovery.
If no blur point: X.
If recovery requires prism of the opposite base as the vergence measured then record as a minus value.

Example, BD/RE: 2/-1.

If limits of prism bar are exceeded then record > max prism value measured.

For example,

At 6 m	BI: X/12/8	BU/RE: 3/1
	BO: 16/22/18	BD/RE: 3/1
At 33 cm	BI: 10/18/14	BU/RE: 3/1
	BO: 28/34/30	BD/RE: 3/1

BI base-in, BO base-out, BU base-up, BD base-down.

Expected findings

	Distance (range Δ)	Near (range Δ)
Negative (BI)		
Blur	X	6 - 10
Break	6 - 12	12 - 18
Recovery	4 - 8	8 - 14
Positive (BO)		
Blur	12 - 16	20 - 28
Break	18 - 22	26 - 34
Recovery	14 - 18	22 - 30

SECTION 7 CONTACT LENSES

Chapter 63 One position keratometer

Chapter 64 Two position keratometer

Chapter 65 Upper lid eversion

Chapter 66 Slit-lamp calibration using patient's closed eye and general set up

Chapter 67 External and anterior eye examination using direct illumination

Chapter 68 Corneal examination using direct illumination

Chapter 69 Corneal examination using indirect and retroillumination

Chapter 70 Corneal examination using specular reflection

Chapter 71 Fluorescein staining

Chapter 72 Using a Wratten 12 filter

Chapter 73 Tear meniscus evaluation

Chapter 74 Soft contact lens insertion

Chapter 75 Soft lens fit assessment

Chapter 76 Soft contact lens removal

Chapter 77 Gas permeable lens insertion

Chapter 78 Gas permeable lens fit assessment

Chapter 79 Gas permeable lens removal

Chapter 63 One position keratometer

Introduction
This instrument measures the curvature of the central cornea over 3-6 mm.

Use
It is used to assess the curvature, power, and toricity of the cornea, as well as the presence of any corneal distortion. The two types of keratometer are one-position and two-position. They differ in the way that the system of 'doubling' is used to measure the separation of mire images. Doubling helps to counteract rapid eye movements that would otherwise make taking the measurement very difficult.

One-position keratometers use variable doubling and their mires have a fixed separation. The separation of the mires is found by varying the doubling power. See Figure 40 below.

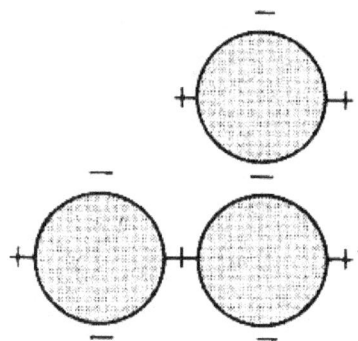

Figure 40 Bausch and Lomb (one-position) mires

Bausch and Lomb (one-position)
There are two sets of fixed mires and two variable doubling devices.
Both principal meridians can be measured at the same time.
For the two vertical circles, the inner minus signs should be overlapping.
For the two horizontal circles, the inner two plus signs should be overlapping.

Procedure
Ensure that the headrest and chinrest of the keratometer have been cleaned and that the patient has removed any glasses or contact lenses.

Adjust the table height so that you and the patient can sit comfortably.
Focus the eyepiece of the keratometer.
Turn the instrument on.
Set the adjustable eyepieces as far clockwise as possible.
Place a piece of white paper in front of the instrument objective to retro-illuminate the target.
Turn the eyepieces clockwise until the target is in focus.
Ask the patient to place their chin on the chinrest and adjust the chinrest height so that the patient's outer canthus is aligned with the mark on the side of the instrument.
Look around the side of the instrument and roughly align the barrel with the patient's right eye (by moving the instrument up, down, left, or right) so that a reflection of the mires appears the patient's cornea.
Instruct the patient to look at the reflection of their own eye in the barrel.
Adjust the power wheel(s) until the mires as close as possible to their aligned position.

If the instrument is one-position there will be two power wheels so that both meridians are measured simultaneously.
Rotate the instrument until the mires are aligned.
Make any further necessary adjustment with the power wheel for optimum alignment.
Repeat for the left eye.

Hints and tips
If the astigmatism is irregular, the meridians may not be 90 degrees apart.
Targets may need to be re-centred and refocused throughout the procedure
The integrity of the tear film can also be assessed by observing the condition of the mires
Sometimes the power of a meridian will fall out of the power range of the instrument
In this case, place a + 1.25 DS in front of the instrument objective lens to extend the steep end of the range, and use a – 1.00 DS lens to extend the flat end of the range
This may be necessary for keratoconic patients
Different instruments may provide different results for the same cornea
This is because the area of cornea used and the refractive index used for calibration varies for different instruments.

Recording findings
Bausch and Lomb RE 7.45 along 150, LE 7.80 along 60.

Chapter 64 Two position keratometer

Introduction
This technique measures the curvature of the central cornea over 3 – 6 mm.

Use
It is used to assess the curvature, power, and toricity of the cornea, as well as the presence of any corneal distortion. The two types of keratometer are one-position and two-position. They differ in the way that the system of 'doubling' is used to measure the separation of mire images. Doubling helps to counteract rapid eye movements that would otherwise make taking the measurement very difficult.

Javal-Schiötz (two-position)
The middle pair of images should be brought together until they just touch. See Figure 41 below.
The instrument may need to be rotated to get the best 'fit'.
Once the first meridian has been measured, the instrument must be rotated by 90 degrees for the second measurement.

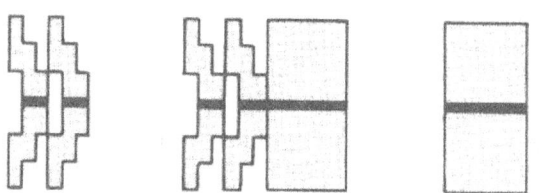

Figure 41 Javal-Schiötz (two-position) mires

Zeiss
The middle pair of images should be superimposed. See Figure 42 below.
The instrument may need to be rotated to get the best 'fit'.
Once the first meridian has been measured, the instrument will need to be rotated by 90 degrees for the second measurement.

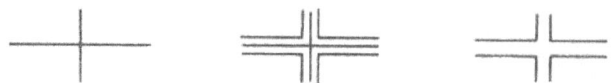

Figure 42 Zeiss mires

Procedure

Ensure that the headrest and chinrest of the keratometer have been cleaned and that the patient has removed any glasses or contact lenses.
Adjust the table height so that you and the patient can sit comfortably.
Focus the eyepiece of the keratometer.
Turn the instrument on.
Set the adjustable eyepieces as far clockwise as possible.
Place a piece of white paper in front of the instrument objective to retro-illuminate the target.
Turn the eyepieces clockwise until the target is in focus.
Ask the patient to place their chin on the chinrest and adjust the chinrest height so that the patient's outer canthus is aligned with the mark on the side of the instrument.
Look around the side of the instrument and roughly align the barrel with the patient's right eye (by moving the instrument up, down, left, or right) so that a reflection of the mires appears the patient's cornea.
Instruct the patient to look at the reflection of their own eye in the barrel.
Adjust the power wheel(s) until the mires as close as possible to their aligned position.
If the instrument is one-position there will be two power wheels so that both meridians are measured simultaneously.
If the instrument is two-position there will be one power wheel and the instrument will have to be rotated by 90 degrees for the second meridian.
Rotate the instrument until the mires are aligned.
Make any further necessary adjustment with the power wheel for optimum alignment.
Repeat for the left eye.

Hints and tips

If the astigmatism is irregular, the meridians may not be 90 degrees apart.
Targets may need to be re-centred and refocused throughout the procedure.
The integrity of the tear film can also be assessed by observing the condition of the mires.
Sometimes the power of a meridian will fall out of the power range of the instrument. In this case, place a + 1.25 DS in front of the instrument objective lens to extend the steep end of the range, and use a − 1.00 DS lens to extend the flat end of the range. This may be necessary for keratoconic patients.
Different instruments may provide different results for the same cornea.
This is because the area of cornea used and the refractive index used for calibration varies for different instruments.

Recording findings

Javal-Schiötz RE 8.05 along 90, LE 8.10 along 180.

Chapter 65 Upper lid eversion

Introduction
Lid eversion allows observation of the palpebral conjunctiva of the upper lid.

Use
It is useful to evert the lids and exam the palpebral conjunctiva using the slit lamp prior to fitting a patient with contact lenses to establish a baseline. It is also indicated if the patient has a red eye or if the patient's symptoms suggest that there may be a foreign body under the upper lid.

Procedure
Set the magnification to 6 - 10X, and the illumination arm to 30 degrees temporal with the system coupled.
Set the illumination level to medium – high and the slit beam width to a medium – wide parallelepiped.
Ask the patient to put their chin on the chin rest with the forehead firmly pressed forward and make sure that the outer canthus is aligned with the mark on the side of the instrument.
Have a clean cotton swab ready.
Advise the patient that this part of the examination might feel unusual but it won't hurt.
Ask the patient to look down.
Using thumb and index finger grasp the patient's upper lid margin and pull gently down and away from the globe.
Using the free hand, insert the cotton swab at the posterior margin of the upper lid (the lid crease).
Press down with the swab while pulling the lid upward and then back against the superior orbital rim.
Remove the cotton swab.
Continue to press the lid against the superior orbital rim and use the slit lamp to exam the tarsal conjunctiva.
Scan the superior palpebral conjunctiva, looking for elevations, foreign bodies or injected blood vessels.
Return the upper lid to its normal position once the examination is complete
When appropriate repeat for the other eye when.

Hints and tips
When pulling the lid margin down and away from the globe make a smooth swift movement, the procedure will be quicker and more comfortable for the patient.
Some upper lid elevations only become apparent using blue light and fluorescein staining.

Recording findings
R upper lid large papillae present.
L upper lid clear and smooth.

Expected findings
R upper lid large papillae present.
L upper lid clear and smooth.

Chapter 66 Slit-lamp calibration using patient's eye and general set up

Introduction
The slit lamp biomicroscope, usually referred to as the slit lamp, is essentially a simple and generally under-used piece of equipment. Although slit lamps vary considerably depending on the manufacturer, there are a number of components common to all slit lamps.

It consists of an illumination system and binocular microscope observation system mounted on a movable platform. Correct alignment of the illumination and observation systems will allow co-incidental focus of the slit beam and microscope. As the relative angle between the slit beam and the microscope is varied, a view of the ocular features can be obtained. The illumination system is a short focus projector, projecting an image of the illuminated slit aperture on to the eye. This part of the system is flexible to allow various sizes and shapes of the slit beam. The slit beam height and width can be adjusted. The angle of the slit beam can be varied from zero degrees in the straight-ahead position, to 90 degrees temporally and nasally with respect to the patient. The click stop changes the position of the reflecting mirror to alter the angle of the beam with respect to the viewing system. When the mirror is 'in click stop', the focus of the slit beam will be co-incident with the focus of the viewing system. When 'out of click stop' the slit beam and viewing system are not co-incident; this feature of the slit lamp can be used to produce indirect and retro-illumination and sclerotic scatter. A rheostat is incorporated to allow changes in the intensity of the illumination and the lamp housing can also be rotated. Neutral density (changes intensity but not colour of the slit beam), cobalt blue (used in conjunction with fluorescein) and red free (green) filters, and occasionally a diffuser are included in the design of most slit lamps.

The observation system consists of a binocular microscope with parallel or convergent eyepieces. Generally magnification from 10X to 40X can be achieved by varying the eyepiece and objective lenses of the microscope. Magnification can be adjusted in a stepwise or continuous fashion when a zoom system is fitted. A focusing joystick and a vertical control knob allow movement of the microscope in the x, y, and z meridians relative to the patient positioned in the head frame.

Use
Optometrists are involved in the examination and care of patients with diabetes, cataract, glaucoma, anterior segment disease such as blepharitis, dry eye, seasonal and contact lens associated conjunctivitis as well as foreign body removal and contact lens fitting and aftercare. Accurate slit lamp evaluation is critical in the

differential diagnosis and correct management of patients with abnormal ocular conditions. The slit lamp techniques described in this chapter will assist the eye-care practitioner in providing the correct management for the patient. It is usual practice to examine the eye in an anterior to posterior sequence and generally in the following order: lashes and lids, conjunctiva, sclera, tear layer, cornea, anterior chamber, iris and lens and anterior vitreous. Slit lamp techniques for investigating the posterior vitreous and retina require auxiliary lenses and these procedures are described in Section 3 Post refraction.

Procedure
General slit lamp set up:
- ➢ Prior to using the slit lamp it is important to spend one or two minutes to make sure that it is set up to provide ease of use and comfort for the patient and practitioner.
- ➢ Repeating this procedure for each patient will allow the maximum amount of clinical information to be gathered in a reasonable period of time.

The following applies to all slit lamp procedures:
The patient is examined without spectacle or contact lens correction in place unless the examination is part of contact lens fitting or aftercare.
Dim room illumination.
Clean the forehead rest and the chin rest with an alcohol or chlorhexidine wipe.
As the patient to lean forward and place their chin on the chin rest and head against the support bar.
Adjust the table height and the chin rest of the slit lamp so that the patient is comfortable and that the outer canthus is aligned with the demarcation line on the upright support of the head rest; this allows maximum play on the vertical height adjustment.
Focus the oculars in turn on the patient's lashes with their eyes closed; focus each ocular by closing one eye at a time and rotating the eyepiece; begin with the eyepiece on the highest plus setting (as far anti-clockwise as possible) and rotate it clockwise until the image just clears.
Set the pupillary distance and make sure that binocular single vision is present.
Remove all filters and set the magnification to its lowest setting, usually x10, as the field of view is maximized by using a low magnification setting.
Check that the illumination and observation systems are coupled i.e. click stop is in.
The joystick/elevation knob may be separate controls or a single control and are found on the base of the instrument; the joystick controls the forward movement, and therefore the focus; the elevation knob controls the height of the microscope.
During a routine slit lamp examination the right eye is usually examined first, followed by the left eye.

Chapter 67 External and anterior eye examination using direct illumination

Introduction
Slit lamp examination of the lids, lashes, conjunctiva, sclera and cornea is important during contact lens fitting and aftercare and for those patients when symptoms or signs suggest the problem may lie with these ocular structures.

Diffuse illumination
This refers to a wide beam that is directed obliquely for general scanning with low magnification in order to maximise the field of view. It is not necessary to have a neutral density filter in place although this may be useful if the patient is photosensitive.

Slit lamp set up
- Coupled
- 30 to 60 degrees beam angle
- 3-4 mm beam width
- Maximum beam height
- No filter
- Medium illumination
- 10X magnification.

Procedure
Position the microscope directly in front of the eye, with the beam at an angle of 60 degrees, and the illumination system and focus on the temporal part of the eye.
Ask the patient to look along the side of the slit lamp:
When examining the patient's right eye the practitioners left ear could be used as a fixation target.
The red fixation light that is attached to most modern slit lamps can be used to move the eye under investigation into any required position.
Use the joystick to scan along the lower lid of the closed eye.
Scan across to the midline and then swing the beam across to the nasal part of the eye and scan back across to the midline.
The procedure should be repeated for the closed upper lid.
Lower and upper lid margins should also be examined with the eye open.
The lower bulbar and palpebral conjunctiva, sclera and cornea can be examined on the open eye by retracting and everting the lower lid with a forefinger.
The patient should be informed of contact prior to touching any part of the eye.
Conjunctiva, sclera and cornea between the lids and then the area beneath the upper lid can be examined in a similar manner.

The upper lid will have to be retracted in order to view the upper bulbar conjunctiva, sclera and cornea.

Hints and tips
Because the beam width is wide and the light is bright some patients may find this technique uncomfortable and it may be necessary to place a neutral density filter between the illumination and the patient.
This can be achieved in most slit lamps by 'dialling in the filter' within the illumination system or by manually flipping a filter over the bulb.
The intensity of the beam can be reduced without sacrificing clarity of view for the examiner.
Novice observers often
Do not realise that the beam is out of click stop and cannot focus the illumination directly on the eye.
Use too high an illumination with can be uncomfortable for the patient and result in 'washing out' features of interest with too much light.
Use too high a magnification which results in loss of perspective of relative structures and a tendency to over interpret normal findings as abnormal.
It is important to shift the illumination arm from one side of the eye to the other when the corneal apex is reached in order to obtain an adequate view of all aspects of the anterior segment.

Recording findings
Diffuse illumination is used to observe the lids and lashes in order to detect the presence and to determine:
Type of blepharitis
Red/pink or crusty lid margins
Meibomian gland dysfunction
Internal and external hordeolum
Lesions that may be neoplastic.
Areas of interest can be further examined by increasing the magnification and narrowing the beam.
Bulbar and palpebral conjunctiva can be investigated with a narrower beam for conjunctival follicles and papillae, hyperaemia and injection, and any evidence of mucus or discharge.
This aids in the differential diagnosis of:
Bacterial, viral, and allergic conjunctivitis
Degenerative lesions of the conjunctiva such as pingeculae and pterygia can also be evaluated and monitored for change.
The sclera can be examined for redness, discoloration, thinning and traumatic damage.
Differential diagnosis between conjunctival and scleral inflammation can be made.
The cornea can be assessed for gross abnormalities due to trauma, oedema or ulcer.

Chapter 68 Corneal examination using direct illumination

Introduction
Slit lamp examination of the cornea is important whenever the anterior segment is assessed. Direct illumination refers to the focusing of the light beam and the microscope in the same area. It does not refer to the coaxial placement of the light source with the microscope. The parallelepiped and optical section are two commonly used types of direct illumination.

Use
The parallelepiped illuminates a three-dimensional corneal area and is effective for detecting a range of lesions. An optic section illuminates a two dimensional area of tissue that is viewed obliquely and is used to localise the depth of lesions. It is used to examine the cornea and in particular to determine the depth of any compromise. The procedure is particularly useful for assessing the area and depth of a corneal abrasion simultaneously, especially when fluorescein has been instilled.

Slit lamp set up for a parallelepiped
- Coupled
- 60 degrees beam angle
- 1-2 mm beam width
- Maximum beam height
- No filter
- Medium illumination
- 10-16X magnification
- Use the joystick to sharply focus the microscope and the parallelepiped simultaneously.

Procedure
The parallelepiped produces a three-dimensional section of the cornea and is useful for the initial examination.
Starting at the temporal limbus, use the joystick to focus the parallelepiped on the inferior of the cornea.
Keep the cornea in focus while scanning across to the nasal limbus.
The lower lid may need to be retracted to view this part of the cornea
Repeat this for the central cornea by scanning form the temporal to nasal limbus and then again for the superior cornea.
The upper lid may need to be retracted to view this area.

Hint and tips
Start with the beam totally extinguished and then slowly open up the beam width adjustor until a thin beam appears.
Continue opening up the adjustor until the beam width is approximately 2mm.
The beam will now have the shape of a parallelepiped.

Recording findings
R cornea clear, L cornea abrasion 7 o'clock extending to corneal apex.

Expected findings
R cornea clear, L cornea clear.

Slit lamp set up for an optic section
- Coupled
- 60 degrees beam angle
- Beam width nearly extinguished
- Maximum beam height
- No filter
- Medium illumination
- 10-16X magnification
- Use the joystick to sharply focus the microscope and the optic section simultaneously.

Procedure
The procedure is the same as parallelepiped illumination except that the beam width is narrowed until it is almost extinguished.
The optic section is sharply focused to localize opacities or staining to a specific corneal layer.
To thoroughly assess the cornea the technique should be repeated with the light source positioned nasally and temporally.

See Figure 43 for an example of an optic section through a healthy cornea.

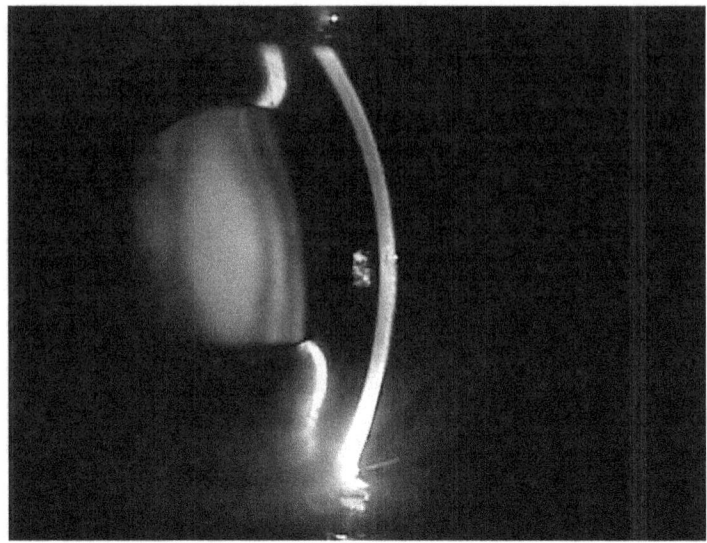

Figure 43 Optic section through a healthy cornea.

Hints and tips
Start with the beam totally extinguished.
Slowly open up the beam width adjustor until a thin beam appears.
Continue opening up the adjustor until the beam width is approximately 0.5 mm.

Recording findings
R cornea abrasion at 7 o'clock on limbus, down to stromal level, L cornea clear.

Expected findings
R cornea clear, L cornea clear.

Chapter 69 Corneal examination using indirect and retroillumination

Introduction
Slit lamp examination of the cornea is important whenever the anterior segment is assessed.

The microscope is focused on an area immediately adjacent to the illuminated tissue. When viewed with direct illumination fine structures, such as neovascularisation, can be 'washed out' and missed due to the high intensity of the direct slit beam.

See Figure 44 for an example of a corneal abnormality illuminated with indirect illumination.

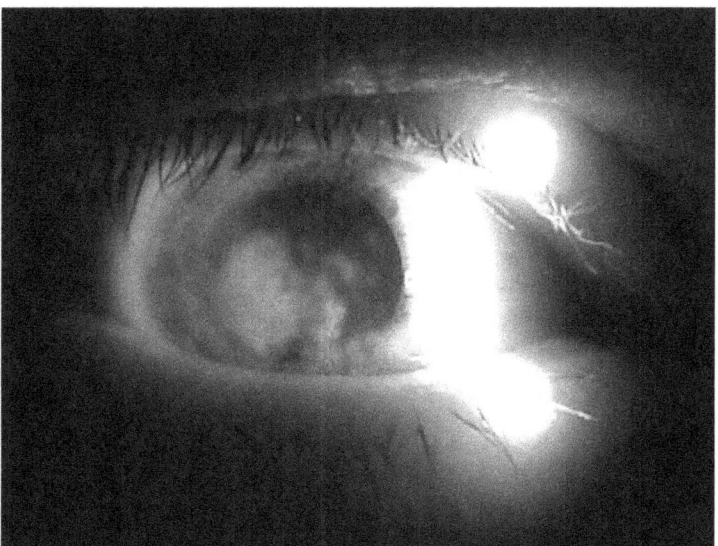

Figure 44 Corneal abnormality illuminated with indirect illumination.

Slit lamp set up
- Coupled or decoupled
- 60 degrees beam angle
- 1 mm beam width
- Maximum beam height
- No filter

- Medium illumination
- 10-16X magnification
- For the right eye adjust the microscope so that the beam is focused to the left of the lesion and change the point of regard to the lesion.

Use
This technique is useful for observing corneal neovascularisation and non-opaque corneal lesions such as microcysts and finger print lines, which are a component of epithelial basement membrane dystrophy. They appear as sinuous, concentric refractile lines.

Procedure
Indirect viewing can be achieved by having the click stop in and looking down the observation system just to the side of the direct beam with the direct beam placed adjacent to the area of interest.
Alternatively with the click stop out, the observation system can be lined up directly with the lesion and the illumination positioned just to the side of it.

Hints and tips
With the click stop in the novice tends to look at the direct beam and miss structures illuminated indirectly.
With the click stop out the inexperienced practitioner often places the illumination out of view of the observation system and features are under-illuminated and thus missed.

Retro-illumination
Light is reflected off the anterior surface of the iris or the retina as the cornea is focused. Opacities will be back lit and appear black due to absorption of the reflected light.

Use
The degree of light absorption will vary with the density of the lesion and therefore a dense corneal opacity will appear black with retroillumination. This technique may be used for the detection, location and assessment of corneal opacities such as ulcers, the detection of fine epithelial and endothelial changes, keratic precipitates and small blood vessels. Pigment derived from the iris may become deposited on the rear surface of the cornea in a characteristic spindle or delta shape.

Slit lamp set up
- Coupled or decoupled
- 60 degrees beam angle
- 1 mm beam width parallelepiped
- Maximum beam height
- No filter
- Medium illumination
- 10-16x magnification.

Procedure
Adjust the microscope so that the corneal lesion is in focus and positioned in front of light reflected off the anterior surface of the iris or the retina.
Alternatively the beam may be moved out of click stop so that the cornea is viewed in light reflected off iris that is not directly behind the corneal area of interest.

Hints and tips
Focus the slit lamp on the cornea and not on the structure that is reflecting light.
Move the light beam until the reflected light illuminates the area of corneal interest.

Recording findings
R cornea 1mm limbal ulcer at 6 o'clock, L cornea neovascularisation between 5 and 6 o'clock.

Expected findings
R cornea clear, L cornea clear.

Chapter 70 Corneal examination using specular reflection

Introduction
Specular reflection is a difficult technique for the novice. Furthermore, it is of limited use during clinical evaluation because of the low magnification available on most slit lamps and the small area of corneal endothelium that can be viewed at one time.

Use
Assessment of the corneal endothelium when symptoms or signs suggest the possibility of corneal endothelial dysfunction.

Slit lamp set up
- Click stop in
- 1-2 mm beam width
- Maximum beam height
- No filter
- Medium illumination
- 10-16x magnification.

Procedure
Use the joystick to focus the microscope and the parallelepiped simultaneously. Adjust the angle of the illumination arm until the slit beam intersects the reflection of the light filament on the cornea. At this point the angle of reflection will be equal to the incident angle of light. An area of bright glare from the front surface of the cornea will be visible through one eyepiece only.
Increase the magnification to x40 at least.
Adjust the focus of the slit lamp so it is sharply focussed on the corneal endothelium. Look for the mosaic pattern of endothelial cells.

Hints and tips
Keep the room lights low.
Sharp focus on the corneal endothelium is crucial.
Move the observation system and readjust the illumination arm to observe other areas of the corneal endothelium.

Recordings
R endothelial blebs L endothelial blebs.

Expected findings
R regular mosaic pattern L regular mosaic pattern.

Chapter 71 Fluorescein staining

Introduction
Ophthalmic dyes are used when slit lamp evaluation of the cornea indicates that the corneal epithelium may be disrupted. This procedure is also indicated when the patient has signs or symptoms suggesting corneal disease. Slit lamp assessment of the cornea is greatly enhanced with the use of staining agents. Fluorescein is an orange dye that fluoresces green when illuminated with a cobalt filter. Areas of corneal or conjunctival epithelial loss will exhibit fluorescein dye uptake and will appear bright green. This positive fluorescein staining will help to identify the extent and distribution of epithelial loss.

Use
The extent and distribution of this staining will be dependent upon the cause of the epithelial disruption. Mucus or epithelial debris in the tear film will also stain brightly with fluorescein. Areas of epithelial elevation cause thinning of the fluorescein-stained tear layer. These areas will appear as black spots within the tear film and are said to exhibit negative fluorescein staining and present as persistent black spots in contrast to the dry spots of tear break-up, which transiently appear within the tear layer as the blink reflex is suppressed.

Fluorescein staining is assessed whenever epithelial loss is suspected, such as following corneal or conjunctival trauma, contact lens removal, gonioscopy, or foreign body removal and to assess corneal involvement secondary to conjunctival, lid, lash and lacrimal disorders. Fluorescein staining will help to assess areas of corneal epithelial elevation as occurs in a healing corneal abrasion or recurrent corneal erosion, in microcystic corneal oedema, and in geographic mapping areas of epithelial basement membrane dystrophy. The elevated epithelium causes a thinning of the precorneal tear film to produce black areas within the tear layer fluorescence. Fluorescein dye will pool in the normal topographical undulations of the bulbar and palpebral conjunctiva. On the bulbar conjunctiva this pooling of dye will appear as a subtle cross hatching effect. On the palpebral conjunctiva, the fluorescein will pool around focal elevations of this tissue and will accentuate the appearance of palpebral conjunctival follicles and papillae. In addition to this normally observed pooling effect, the conjunctiva will also exhibit frank fluorescein staining when the epithelium is disrupted. During dry eye management the amount of staining can be monitored to gauge success with treatment.

Slit lamp set up for fluorescein staining
- Click stop in
- 60 degree beam angle
- 3-4 mm beam width

- Maximum beam height
- Cobalt filter
- Maximum illumination
- 6-10X magnification.

Procedure
The dye-impregnated end of a sterile fluorescein strip should be wetted with one drop of sterile saline.
With the patient looking up the strip should be gently touched against the lower bulbar conjunctiva of the right eye for one second and then removed.
It is important to use the blunt or flat side of the strip and not the edge as this may cut the conjunctiva or cornea in a similar way that paper can cut the skin of a finger.
Using the same strip repeat this procedure for the left eye.
If there is evidence of anterior segment disease in one eye, use the strip on the uninvolved eye first or use separate strips for each eye.
Allow the fluorescein dye to diffuse for approximately 30 seconds.
Scan the cornea and bulbar conjunctiva for areas of dye uptake that appear bright green.
To assess the palpebral conjunctiva, retract the lower lid as the patient looks up and also evert the upper lid.

Hints and tips
Make sure that the beam is in the click position and that the patient's eyes are in primary gaze.
Fluorescein staining should be performed prior to the instillation of topical ophthalmic anaesthetic solution since corneal staining may be induced.
That portion of the bulbar conjunctiva that is touched with the vital dye strip will stain densely and should not be misinterpreted as an abnormality.
After placing one drop of saline on to the fluorescein strip shake the strip over a sink or wastebasket to remove the excess.
The strip should now be moist and glisten when held to the light.
Introducing too much fluorescein in to the eye will result in subtle staining being obscured by an intense green background colour.
It is best to touch the strip to the inferior bulbar conjunctiva as applying it to the superior bulbar conjunctiva runs the risk of touching the cornea if the patient exhibits a Bell's reflex, and the eye rotates upwards.
Prior to examination allow the fluorescein dye to drain for 30 seconds.
With significant corneal epithelial disruption, the anterior chamber should be evaluated prior to the instillation fluorescein.
Fluorescein may penetrate through the cornea into the anterior chamber and produce a green tinged-flare that may be misinterpreted as protein in the anterior chamber.
Novice clinicians often think that the presence of staining will be more easily detected when lots of fluorescein is instilled.
This is incorrect as excess fluorescein often masks the presence of subtle staining, when there is so much fluorescein present that the pathological stain is shrouded by the physiological stain of the tears.
This is especially true when fluorescein is applied from a Minim.

These should only be used in the assessment of the fit of a scleral lens and should never be used in the assessment of staining.

Fluorescein is a dye and like most dyes it will stain clothes and skin and care needs to be taken not to splash any on to clothes or skin.

When the fluorescein has been applied to the eye immediately wrap the strip in its sleeve and dispose.

Recording findings

R cornea clear, L superficial punctate staining superior cornea between 10 and 2 o' clock.

Expected findings

R cornea clear, L cornea clear.

Chapter 72 Using a Wratten 12 barrier filter

Introduction
Slit lamp fluorescein exams can be enhanced with this yellow barrier filter by filtering excess blue light, reflected from the front surfaces of the eye.

Use
The contrast between areas of intact and areas of broken tear film is enhanced when excess blue light is prevented from entering the microscope observation system of the slit lamp. Timely identification of areas of broken tear film means that tear break up time can be more accurately determined.

Enhancing the contrast at of the tear meniscus where the inner margin of the lower lid meets the cornea means that the upper and lower borders of the tear meniscus are more clearly delineated leading to a more accurate measurement of tear meniscus height.

Slit lamp set up
- Instillation of fluorescein
- Blue filter in place
- Maximum illumination
- 10X magnification
- Any form of direct illumination.

Procedure
Wratten 12 filter introduced immediately in front of the objective lens of the microscope observation system.
Look through pre-focussed and aligned eye piece lenses.
Observe tear break up time and/or tear meniscus height.

Chapter 73 Tear meniscus evaluation

Introduction
The tear layer is comprised of the outer lipid layer, middle aqueous layer, and inner mucin layer. The tear film can be stained with fluorescein dye and then observed with the slit lamp for tear break up and tear meniscus height.

In addition to the lacrimal lake in the medial canthal area, strips of tear fluid are located at the posterior margins of both the upper and lower eyelids. This tear strip is wedge or meniscus shaped as it simultaneously contacts the lid margin and the bulbar conjunctiva with the lid in the normal position. The quality of the tear layer can be assessed by inspection of the meniscus with the slit lamp.

Use
Normally the tear meniscus should be 1 mm wide. In patients with dry eye the meniscus may be significantly reduced in size due to the reduced quantities of the aqueous tear component. The resultant concentration of the oily and mucin tear layers may produce significant levels of mucous strands and debris in the tear strip and the tear strip will appear very viscous. The tear strip will frequently exhibit superficial coloured moiré reflections off the outermost oily layer. Excessive tear lipids commonly occur in patients with Meibomian gland over secretion or seborrheic blepharitis. A patient with bacterial conjunctivitis will exhibit exudative debris and mucus in the tear strip. Evaluation of the tear meniscus height during management of dry eye will give an indication of treatment success.

Slit lamp set up
- Coupled
- 60 degree beam angle
- Beam width equivalent to a parallelepiped
- Maximum beam height
- No filter
- Low illumination
- 10-16x magnification.

Procedure
Focus the parallelepiped on the inferior tear strip near the lateral canthus.
Use the joystick to scan across the tear strip, moving nasally and keeping the strip in focus.
At any point the beam may be narrowed to an optic section to assess the depth of the tear meniscus.

Hints and tips
Turning the illumination too high may induce reflex tearing and obscure the viscosity and thinning of the tear meniscus.
The tear meniscus should be evaluated prior to any planned lid eversion of the upper lid as this may result in expression of the Meibomian gland secretions in to the tear strip and will artifactually contribute to the appearance of debris.
Lid eversion may also induce reflex tearing.

Recording findings
R tear meniscus 0.5 mm, L tear meniscus 0.5 mm.

Expected findings
R tear meniscus >1mm, L tear meniscus > 1mm.

Chapter 74 Soft contact lens insertion

Introduction
Practitioners must be able to insert and remove soft contact lenses in order to fit new patients, and in the event that a contact lens patient presents with a problem.

Use
New patients, as well as those with poor manual dexterity will be unable to insert and remove contact lenses themselves.

Procedure
Wash hands and dry with a lint-free towel.
Take the lens out of its container and make sure that it is positioned the right way out on finger.
Inspect the lens for defects, tears, or debris.
If defects or tears are present, replace the lens.
If debris is present, rinse the lens with sterile saline.
It is good practice to rinse a new lens with saline even if it appears clean.
Place the lens on the tip of the index finger of the dominant hand.
Make sure that this finger is dry as a hydrophilic lens tends to stick to the finger rather that the patient's eye.
Ask the patient to look up and place the index finger or thumb of the other hand on the lid margin of the patient's upper lid.
Pull the lid back and hold it firmly against the upper brow.
Ask the patient to look up and place the middle or fourth finger of your dominant hand on the lower lid.
Pull the lid down and hold firmly.
Gently apply the lens to the eye in one of three ways
With the patient looking up, place the lens on the inferior sclera.
With the patient looking temporally, place the lens on the temporal sclera.
With the patient looking straight ahead, place the lens on the cornea.
Keep hold of the lids and ask the patient to look straight ahead to centre the lens.
If it does not centre, keep hold of the lids and ask the patient to look up, down, left, and right.
This should help the lens to settle on the cornea.
Gently release the upper and lower lids.

Hints and tips
Make sure that the fingernails are short and clean.
Remember to explain to new patients that the lids will have to be held firmly.

Chapter 75 Soft contact lens fit assessment

Introduction
Soft contact lens fit assessment determines whether or not a contact lens is fitting well and is suitable for the patient.

Use
Adequate fitting is necessary for optimal vision and comfort, and to minimise the risk of complications.

Procedure
The slit lamp should be set up that so that you and the patient are comfortable.
Set the magnification to 6 or 10X, and the illumination arm to 30 degrees temporal.
Set the illumination level to medium – high and the slit beam width to a medium parallelepiped.
Ask the patient to put their chin on the chin rest and make sure that the outer canthus is aligned with the mark on the side of the instrument.
Ask the patient to look straight ahead.
Move the slit beam from the temporal to nasal lens edge and observe the lens position and corneal coverage.
Ask the patient to blink and then observe any induced lens movement.
Observe this movement at 6 o'clock, if you can see the edge at that position. If not, observe the movement at the temporal and nasal lens edge nearest to the lower lid.
This process can be repeated two or three times.
To observe vertical lag, instruct the patient to look up and note how much the lens moves down.
While the patient is looking up, ask him/her to blink two or three times and observe the amount of movement induced.
As the patient to look straight ahead, and then to the right.
Note the amount of lateral lag movement induced and repeat with the patient looking to the left.
Ask the patient to look straight ahead again and explain that you are about to touch their lower lid.
Perform the push-up test by using the patient's lower lid to push up on the inferior edge of the contact lens.
Note the ease or difficulty with which the lens moves upwards.
If assessing the fit of a toric lens, make a note of its rotational orientation and stability.
Ask the patient to look straight ahead and locate the orientation markings on the toric lens.
Measure or estimate the amount and direction of rotation of the markings from their intended position.

Ask the patient to blink and observe the rotational stability of the lens markings. Record the lens position, corneal coverage, blink and lag movement, and push-up movement observed.
If assessing a toric lens, record the rotational orientation and stability of the lens.

Hints and tips
If there is a graticule on the slit lamp, use it to help estimate the amount of movement of the lens.

Recording findings
For a well-fitting spherical soft lens, an example record may read:
Lens position and coverage: central and full.
Blink movement: 1 mm in primary gaze (straight ahead) and 1.5 mm in up gaze
Lag movement: 1.5 mm in up gaze and lateral gaze
Optimal push-up.
For a well-fitting soft toric lens, an example record may read:
Lens position and coverage: central and full.
Blink movement: 1mm in primary gaze, 1.5 mm in up gaze.
Lag movement: 1.5 mm in up gaze and lateral gaze.
Push-up movement: optimal.
Rotational orientation: 5 degrees clockwise.
Rotational stability: no rotation on blink.
Consider drawing diagrams to indicate lens position and rotation.

Chapter 76 Soft contact lens removal

Introduction
Practitioners must be able to insert and remove soft contact lenses in order to fit new patients, and in the event that a contact lens patient presents with a problem.

Use
New patients, as well as those with poor manual dexterity will be unable to insert and remove contact lenses themselves.

Procedure
Ask the patient to look down and use the non-dominant hand to hold the upper lid firmly against the brow.
Ask the patient to look up and use the middle or fourth finger of the dominant hand to firmly retract the lower lid.
Place the index finger of the dominant hand on the inferior portion of the lens and pull it downwards towards the sclera.
While the lens is displaced, pinch it off the cornea with the index finger and thumb.
Alternatively, ask the patient to look nasally and slide the lens temporally until it comes out, or gathers at the outer canthus from where it can be can be gently pinched off.

Hints and tips
Make sure that the fingernails are short and clean.
Remember to explain to new patients that the lids will have to be held firmly.

Chapter 77 Gas permeable lens insertion

Introduction
Practitioners must be able to insert and remove gas permeable contact lenses in order to fit new patients, and in the event that a contact lens patient presents with a problem.

Use
New patients, as well as those with poor manual dexterity will be unable to insert and remove contact lenses themselves.

Procedure
Wash hands and dry with a lint-free towel.
Take the lens out of its container and make sure that it is positioned the right way out on finger.
Inspect the lens for defects, tears, or debris.
If defects are present, replace the lens.
If debris is present, rinse the lens with sterile saline.
It is good practice to rinse a new lens with saline even if it appears clean.
Add a drop of wetting solution to each side of the lens.
Place the lens on the tip of the index finger of the dominant hand.
Ask the patient to look up and place the index finger or thumb of the other hand on the lid margin of the patient's upper lid.
Pull the lid back and hold it firmly against the upper brow.
Ask the patient to look up and place the middle or fourth finger of your dominant hand on the lower lid.
Pull the lid down and hold firmly.
With the patient looking straight ahead, place the lens on the cornea.
Gently release the upper and lower lids.

Hints and tips
Make sure that the fingernails are short and clean.
Remember to explain to new patients that the lids will have to be held firmly.

Chapter 78 Gas permeable lens fit assessment

Introduction
Gas permeable lens fit assessment determines whether a contact lens is fitting well and is suitable for the patient.

Use
Adequate fitting is necessary for optimal vision and comfort, and to minimise the risk of complications. The fit of a gas permeable lens (GP) can be assessed with a slit lamp and a Burton lamp.

Slit lamp set up
- The slit lamp should be set up that so that you and the patient are comfortable.
- Set the magnification to 6 or 10X, and the illumination arm to 30 degrees temporal.
- Set the illumination level to medium – high and the slit beam width to full.
- Place the yellow filter over the objective end of the slit lamp.

Wet a fluorescein strip with sterile saline and shake off the excess saline.
Instil a minimum amount of fluorescein onto the inferior or superior bulbar conjunctiva.
To assess the right lens, ask the patient to look straight ahead.
View the contact lens through the eyepieces.

Observe the static lens fit:
- Lens position.
- Corneal position where the lens settles after a blink.
- Fluorescein pattern.
- The amount of fluorescein underneath the lens should be evaluated in the central, mid-peripheral, and peripheral zones of the lens.
- Darker areas indicate 'touch' between the lens and the cornea.
- Green/yellow areas indicate pooling, where there is space between the lens and cornea.
- Green/black areas indicate alignment between the back surface of the contact lens and the cornea.

If the lens is decentred, the fluorescein fit should also be assessed with the lens centred on the cornea.
This can achieved by manipulating the lens with the lids.
Dynamic aspects of the fit can be assessed by asking the patient to blink.

Record the lens position, blink movement, stability, and fluorescein pattern for each eye.

Hints and tips
If there is a graticule on the slit lamp, use it to help estimate the amount of lens movement.

Recording findings
For an acceptable GP lens fit, an example record may read:
Lens position: central
Blink movement: approximately 2 mm
Lens remains central and stable
Fluorescein pattern: central alignment, mid-peripheral bearing, peripheral clearance.

Chapter 79 Gas permeable lens removal

Introduction
Practitioners must be able to insert and remove gas permeable contact lenses in order to fit new patients, and in the event that a contact lens patient presents with a problem.

Use
New patients, as well as those with poor manual dexterity will be unable to insert and remove contact lenses themselves.

Procedure
Ask the patient to look straight ahead.
Place tips of index fingers or thumbs on the patient's lid margins at the superior and inferior lens positions.
Move the lids back so that the margins are just outside the edge of the lens. Make sure that edge of the lid does not roll out or in.
Gently press in onto the lids, and move the lids towards each other until one edge of the lens comes away from the corneal surface.
Continue to move the lids towards each other until the lens is completely removed.
Ask the patient to keep his/her eyes closed until the lens has been removed from the lashes.

Hints and tips
Make sure that fingernails are short and clean.
Explain to new patients that they may feel some discomfort when the lens has been inserted.
It is better to be firm and remove the lens on the first attempt rather than to be too delicate in approach and still not have removed the lens after the third or fourth attempt.

GLOSSARY

A-pattern	Relative increase in exophoria on down gaze, or increase in esophoria on up gaze.
Accommodation	The involuntary ability to adjust the power of the eye by changing the shape of the crystalline lens.
Accommodative spasm	Spasm of the ciliary muscles that may result in pseudomyopia.
Accommodative	A change that provokes an accommodative response, such as the stimulus introduction of a near target.
Afferent pathway	Consists of nerves that carry impulses towards the central nervous system.
Alleviating	Reducing symptoms, e.g. *alleviating or relieving prism* used to relieve symptoms caused by uncompensated heterophoria.
Ametropia	State in which, when the accommodation is relaxed, objects at infinity are not focussed on the retina (see hypermetropia and myopia).
Angle kappa	Angle between the visual axis and the pupillary axis, measured at the nodal point
Angle lambda	Angle between the line of sight formed at the centre of the entrance pupil and the papillary axis.
Anhydrosis	Deficiency or absence of perspiration.
Anisocoria	Unequal pupil sizes.
Anisometropia	The eyes require different refractive corrections.
Anomalous trichromatism	A defect of vision in which the three primary colours are required for colour matching but the proportions of each colour are different to normal trichromatism.
Anterior chamber	Space between the cornea and the iris and anterior lens surface that visible through the pupil. Filled with the aqueous humour.
Anterior segment	Front portion of the eye, including cornea, aqueous humour, ciliary body, and lens.
Applanation tonometry	Flattening of the cornea by pressure, as used in applanation.
Arcus senilis	The appearance of a yellowish-grey lipid ring around the margin of the cornea, most commonly in older people.
Artefactual	Of spurious nature, not naturally present and perhaps the product of the examination technique itself, e.g. the reflection on the fundus photograph was artefactual.
Asthenopia	Eyestrain.
Astigmatism	The unequal curvature of one or more refractive surfaces of the eye, usually the cornea, prevents clear focusing at one point on the retina, resulting in blurred vision. Meridians of greatest and least curvature are at right-angles to each other.
Bifoveal fixation	The object is imaged by both fovea at the same time

Binocular	Both eyes.
Binocular vision	Use of both eyes together.
Bracketing	Process of jumping above and below the final refraction result in decreasing steps to find the final value.
Bruch's membrane	Inner layer of the choroid in contact with the retinal pigment epithelium.
Cataract	Loss of transparency of the crystalline lens.
Cerebrovascular brain, also accident	Blockage or haemorrhage of a blood vessel leading to the known as a stroke
Chiasmal lesion	Lesion of the optic chiasm, which is located above the pituitary gland and is formed by the meeting and partial crossing-over of the optic nerves. The lesion results in a heteronymous hemianopia-type visual field defect
Choroid	Pigmented, highly vascular membrane that is continuous with the iris and lies between the sclera and the retina, functioning to nourish the retina and absorb scattered light
Ciliary body	An annular structure on the inner surface of the anterior wall of the eyeball composed largely of the ciliary muscle and bearing the ciliary processes
Comitancy	There is a constant angle between the two eyes for all positions of gaze when fixating at a fixed distance. Also known as concomitance.
Compensated	Does not give rise to symptoms, e.g. *compensated heterophoria*.
Condensing lens	A lens designed to be used for fundus examination with a biomicroscope, that has a large aperture and short focal length such that as much light as possible is directed towards the retina.
Conjunctival sac	The space bound by the conjunctival membrane between the palpebral (posterior surface of eyelid) and bulbar (anterior face of the sclera) conjunctiva of the eye.
Convergence excess	High esophoria at near associated with relative orthophoric conditions when viewing a distant target, which may be accompanied by asthenopia.
Cornea	The transparent convex anterior portion of the outer fibrous coat of the eyeball that covers the iris and the pupil and is continuous with the sclera.
Corneal reflex	Image caused by reflection of light from the cornea.
Crossed disparity	Fixation disparity induced when the object is closer to the eyes than the point of fixation and so is focused on the temporal retina.
Crystalline lens	A doubly convex, transparent body in the eye, situated behind the iris, that focuses incident light on the retina
Cyl	Lens used to correct astigmatism.
Cyclophoria	Heterophoria in which the visual axes of the eyes tend to rotate outwards (excyclophoria) or inwards (incyclophoria).
Cycloplegia	Paralysis of the ciliary muscles of the eye, resulting in loss of the ability to accommodate.

Cycloplegic drops	Eye drops used to induce cycloplegia, e.g. cyclopentolate.
Decompensation	Failure of a system or organ to carry out its function. For example, failure of the visual system to compensate for heterophoria.
Decibel (dB)	Commonly used to describe light intensities used in visual field testing. A decibel scale is a logarithmic scale in which 10 decibels are equal to 1 log unit, and 20 decibels are equal to 20 log units, and so on. Decibels are used to describe the attenuation of the brightness of a stimulus, such that a 20 dB stimulus is equal to one-tenth the brightness of a 10 dB stimulus.
Deutan	Person who has deuteranopia or deuteranomaly
Deuteranomaly	Type of anomalous trichromatism in which an abnormally high proportion of green is needed when mixing red and green light to match a given yellow. Sensitivity of the retina to green light is deficient. Occurs in 4.6 % of men and 0.35 % of women.
Deuteranopia	Type of dichromatic colour deficiency in which red and green are confused although their apparent brightness is almost the same as in normals. There is a reduced sensitivity to green light. Wavelengths above 498 nm appear yellowish and wavelengths below it appear bluish. Occurs in just over 1 % of men and rarely in women
Dichromatic colour	A defect of vision in which the retina responds to only two of the three vision defect primary colours.
Dioptre	Unit used to quantify the refractive error of a lens or optical system.
Diplopia	Double vision.
Dissociation	Removing the stimulus to fuse, normally by occluding one eye.
Duction	Movement of one eye alone.
Duochrome	Subjective refraction test in which the subject compares the sharpness of black targets on a red background with the sharpness of identical targets on a green background
Ectropion	Outward turning of the eyelid.
Efferent pathway	Consists of nerves that carry impulses away from the central nervous system, towards an effector.
Enophthalmos	Recession of the eyeball within the orbit.
Entrance pupil (eye)	Image of the iris aperture formed by the cornea.
Entropion	Inward turning of the eyelid.
Epicanthus	A fold of skin extending from the eyelid over the inner canthus of the eye.
Epiphora	Overflow of tears due to impairment of outflow.
Esophoria	Tendency for the visual axes to be directed inwards with respect to the fixation target. Nasal movement of the eye when it is occluded.
Esotropia	Strabismus in which the deviating eye(s) turns inwards.

Exophoria	Tendency for the visual axes to be directed outwards with respect to the fixation target. Temporal movement of the eye when it is occluded.
Exotropia	Strabismus in which the deviating eye(s) turns outwards.
External hordeolum	Inflammation of infected eyelash follicles and surrounding sebaceous glands of the lid margin. Also known as a stye.
Extra-ocular muscles	Six small muscles that control the horizontal, vertical, and rotating movements of the eyeball.
Fixate	Focus the eyes on.
Fixation disparity	The retinal images of an object do not fall on corresponding retinal points. If the two images still fall within a certain range (called Panum's area), then the image will still be seen as single.
Fovea	Central, depressed area of the retina, located within the macula, where there are mainly cones and the retina is at its thinnest, that gives rise to highest visual acuity.
Foveal reflex	Reflection of light from the concave surface of the foveal depression of the retina. Seen during ophthalmoscopy, more easily in younger eyes.
Full threshold strategy	Visual field testing strategy in which the threshold luminance value is determined at several points within the visual field and is then compared with age-matched 'normal' values. It is the most accurate way of tracking glaucomatous defects.
Fundus	The interior of the eye, as viewed during ophthalmoscopy, including the retina, retinal blood vessels, optic disc, fovea, and sometimes choroidal vessels.
Gas permeable lens	Hard contact lens that transmits oxygen.
Glaucoma	A group of eye diseases that result in visual field loss, often associated with raised intra-ocular pressure.
Halberg clip	A plastic device that can be clipped onto existing spectacles with two cells for holding trial lenses.
Heterochromia	A difference in coloration in two anatomical structures or two parts of the same structure that are normally alike in colour (*heterochromia* of the iris).
Heterophoria	A tendency for the visual axes not to be directed towards the fixation point. Also known as latent strabismus
Heterotropia	See *strabismus*.
Horner's syndrome	Interruption of the sympathetic nerve supply to the dilator pupillae muscle that can result in ptosis, miosis, enophthalmos, heterochromia, and anhydrosis/flushing of the face.
Hyperopia	Long-sightedness, distant images are focussed behind the retina when the accommodation is relaxed. Younger people may be able to accommodate to bring the focus onto the retina.
Hypertropia	Strabismus in which the deviating eye turns upwards.
Hypopyon	An effusion of pus into the anterior chamber of the eye.
Hypotropia	Strabismus in which the deviating eye turns downwards.

Incomitancy	The angle between the eyes is not constant for all positions of gaze when fixating at a fixed distance. Also known as inconcomitance.
Injected blood vessels	Blood vessels that are visibly distended with blood.
Intraocular pressure	The pressure within the eyeball that gives it a round firm shape and is caused by the aqueous humor and vitreous humour.
Iris	The contractile, circular diaphragm forming the coloured portion of the eye and containing a circular opening, the pupil, in its centre.
Irregular astigmatism	Ocular astigmatism in which the two principle meridians are not at right-angles to each other. Often the result of injury or disease.
Isopters	Contour lines representing the limits of retinal sensitivity to a particular target.
Kinetic perimetry	Assessment of the extent of the visual field with a moving target of fixed luminance.
Latent deviation	See *heterophoria*.
Low vision aids	Appliances used to improve visual function in people with visual loss, e.g., magnifiers.
Luminance	The quantitative measure of brightness of a light source or an illuminated surface, equal to luminous flux per unit solid angle emitted per unit projected area of the source or surface.
Macula	Central part of the retina, centred on the fovea.
Macular oedema	Presence of excessive fluid in or around the cells and tissues of the macula. Results in deterioration of visual acuity.
Maculopathy	Degeneration of the macular area of the retina.
Media opacities	Localised or diffuse loss of transparency of the cornea, aqueous humour, crystalline lens, or vitreous humour.
Meridians	Lines surrounding the surface of the eye and passing through both anterior and posterior poles.
Metamorphopsia	The apparent distortion of an image.
Minutes of arc	Unit of angular distance equal to a 60th of a degree.
Miosis	Excessive constriction of the pupil of the eye, as a result of drugs or disease.
Monocular	One eye.
Monocular cues	Aid judgement of the distance between a distant object and the observer, or the distance between two distant objects, also known as depth perception. This process is more accurate with binocular vision, but possible with monovision.
Mydriasis	Extensive dilation of the pupil.
Mydriatic	Eye drop used to induce mydriasis, e.g. tropicamide.
Myopia	Short-sightedness, distant images are focussed in front of the retina and so appear blurred.
Nasal	Pertaining to the nose, e.g., the lesion is situated *nasal* to the optic disc.

Near add	Difference in spherical power between the distance and near corrections.
Neovascularisation	Growth of new blood vessels, often of abnormal quantity and with negative effects.
Neural retinal rim	Part of the optic disc that contains the neural elements. Situated between the cup and the edge of the disc, and so shaped like a ring-doughnut.
Nonius lines	A pair of lines, one of which is seem by the right eye and the other of which is seen by the left eye. Used in the Mallett fixation disparity test.
Nuclear sclerosis	Age-related loss of transparency or yellowing of the crystalline lens, also known as nuclear cataract.
Nystagmus	Involuntary, repetitive movement of the eye.
Objective angle	Angle of strabismus measured without input from the patient.
Objective test	A test that does not rely on responses from the patient.
Occipital	Pertaining to the occipital bone, at the back and base of the skull.
Occluder	Opaque strip used to cover one eye.
Occlusion	Process of occluding an eye.
Oculocentric	Using the eye as a centre of reference.
Oedema	Presence of excess fluid in or around cells and tissues of the body. Can occur in the conjunctiva, cornea, ciliary body, retina (and specifically macula), and choroids.
Optic cup:disc ratio	Ratio of the horizontal diameter of the physiological optic cup to the horizontal diameter of the optic disc. For example, if the optic cup is half the width of the optic disc, the horizontal ratio would be 0.5.
Optic cup, physiological	Depressed are near the centre of the optic disc, through which the central retinal artery passes. Usually paler in colour than the neural retinal rim.
Optic disc	Region of the fundus where the optic nerve enters the eye. Also known as the optic nerve head.
Optic nerve crescents	A pale, crescent-shaped patch of sclera seen adjacent to the optic disc (congenital, scleral) that occurs when the choroid and retinal pigment epithelium do not reach the disc. Present at birth.
Optic nerve crescents	Crescent seen on the temporal side of the disc in myopia. Result of (myopic) atrophy of the retinal pigment epithelium and choroid.
Orbit	The bony cavity of the skull that contains the eye, also known as eye socket.
Orthophoria	Absence of heterophoria.
Orthoptic eye exercises	Exercises designed to improve anomalies of binocular vision.
Orthotropia	Absence of strabismus.
Palpebral aperture	Space between the eyelid margins when the eye is open.

Palpebral conjunctiva	The part of the conjunctiva lining the posterior surface of the eyelids; continuous with the bulbar conjunctiva and attached to the posterior surfaces of the tarsal plates. Also known as tarsal conjunctiva.
Panum's area	The retinal area over which the image of an object can fall such that the images from both eyes are fused and the subject does not experience diplopia. Its diameter in the fovea is about 5 minutes of arc and it increases towards the periphery.
Papilla	Small, pimple-shaped elevation. Papillae (plural).
Paretic	Experiencing some degree of paralysis.
Phenylephrine	A sympathomimetic drug, used in the form of eye drops to dilate the pupil.
Phi movement	Illusion of movement created when one object disappears and an identical one replaces it in a neighbouring region of the screen. Used to create illusion of movement in films.
Phoropter	A device containing a range of lenses used for refracting the eye during a sight test. Used instead of a trial frame.
Photoreceptors	Light sensitive cells (rods and cones) within the retina.
Phototoxic	Renders cells and tissues susceptible to damage by light.
Pituitary tumour visual	Tumour of the pituitary gland that results in bitemporal field defects.
Posterior chamber	Space between the posterior iris surface and the anterior surface of the lens that is filled with aqueous humour.
Posterior pole	Intersection of the sclera with the geometric axis of the eye, also used to describe the optic disc area of the fundus.
Posterior segment	Posterior portion of the eye, including vitreous humour, retina, optic disc, choroid, and most of the sclera.
Presbyope	Person who is experiencing presbyopia.
Presbyopia	Age-related deterioration of the ability to accommodate.
Primary open angle	Glaucoma in which the angle between the iris and the cornea is open glaucoma and so aqueous humour has access to drainage systems.
Primary position of	Looking straight ahead gaze.
Prism bar	A bar made up of prisms of different strengths that can be held up in front of the patient's eye and used to make measurements of the amount of heterophoria or heterotropia.
Prism dioptre	Unit of prismatic deviation, in which the number one represents a prism that deflects a beam of light a distance of one centimetre on a plane placed normal to the initial direction of the beam and one meter away from the prism.
Prismatic effect	The difference in prismatic effect induced by a pair of spectacle lenses of (differential) different powers when the eyes look in different directions of gaze.
Protan	Person who has protanopia or protanomaly.
Protanomaly	A form of anomalous trichromatism in which an excessive amount of red is required when mixing red and green to

	match a given yellow. Sensitivity to red is diminished. Occurs in around 1 % of men.
Protanopia	A form of dichromatic colour deficiency characterized by defective perception of red and confusion of red with green or bluish green. Below 493 nm all wavelengths appear bluish, whereas above it they all appear yellowish. There is a lack of sensitivity to red or green. Occurs in around 1 % of men.
Proxymetacaine	A local anaesthetic that is used in the form of eye drops to eliminate sensitivity of the surface of the eye.
Pseudomyopia	A condition simulating myopia due to spasm of the ciliary muscles.
Pseudophakic eye	Eye fitted with an intra-ocular lens implant (commonly after cataract surgery).
Pseudostrabismus	Condition in which there appears to be a strabismus (often associated with epicanthus, or a broad nasal bridge in young children), but in which corneal light reflexes are centrally located with respect to the pupil.
Ptosis	Narrowing of the palpebral aperture normally associated with drooping of the upper eyelid, but rarely with elevation of the lower eyelid.
Pupil dilation	Enlargement of the pupil aperture in response to low light levels, or *mydriasis*.
Purkinje images	Images produced by reflection from the optical surfaces of the eye. The first is reflected by the anterior surface of the cornea, the second by the posterior surface of the cornea, the third by the anterior lens surface, and the fourth by the posterior lens surface. Also known as Purkinje-Sanson images.
RAF rule	Rule that is held up to the patient's face and used to measure accommodation and convergence.
Red reflex	Light reflected from the fundus during ophthalmoscopy or retinoscopy that makes the pupil appear red.
Refraction	Process of determining the refractive error of an eye.
Refractive error	The dioptric power of the ametropia of an eye.
Retina	Inner most coat of the posterior part of the eyeball that receives the image produced by the lens, is continuous with the optic nerve, and consists of several layers, one of which contains the rods and cones that are sensitive to light.
Retinal pigment	Pigmented layer of cells that lies between the photoreceptors and epithelium Bruch's membrane within the retina. Functions include absorption of light and regeneration of visual pigment.
Retinoscopy	Objective method of determining refractive error.
Sclera	Dense, white, fibrous membrane that, with the cornea, forms the external covering of the eyeball.
Scotoma	Loss of vision in part of the visual field.
Sensorial dysfunction	Disruption of an impulse that should result in sensation.

Smooth pursuit	Movement of the eye when it is fixating on a moving target.
Soft contact lens	Contact lens made of flexible plastic material that transmits a certain amount of oxygen.
Soft toric lens	Soft contact lens designed to correct astigmatism.
Spot retinoscope	A retinoscope that projects a circular beam of light onto the patient's retina.
Static perimetry	The assessment of the extent of the visual field by presenting a target at different retinal locations. The retinal sensitivity at each location is assessed by altering the size or luminance of the target.
Stereoacuity	The smallest difference in distance between two objects presented to both eyes that can be detected.
Stereopsis	The ability to perceive depth.
Strabismus	Both eyes cannot be directed at the same point at the same time.
Streak retinoscope	A retinoscope that projects a streak of light onto the patient's retina. May be easier to assess astigmatism with this type than with the spot retinoscope.
Subjective test	A test that relies on responses from the patient.
Superior orbital rim	Frontal, superior part of the orbit, formed by the frontal bone.
Suprathreshold strategy	Visual field testing strategy in which stimuli are presented at luminance levels higher than normal threshold values in various locations across the visual field. Targets that are seen indicate normal visual function whereas those not seen indicate areas of decreased visual sensitivity. This technique is generally used for screening.
Systemic hypertension	Arterial disease in which chronic high blood pressure is the primary symptom.
Tarsal conjunctiva	See *palpebral conjunctiva*.
Temporal	Pertaining to the temporal bones, which form the part of the skull that encases the inner ear, e.g., the macula is situated *temporal* to the optic disc.
Threshold	The value of a stimulus that just produces a response.
Tonometry	Measurement of the intra-ocular pressure of the eye.
Toricity	A measure of the difference between the most the curved and least curved meridians of a surface.
Trial lens	Lenses that are placed in the trial frame during refraction of an eye.
Trichromatism	Normal colour vision.
Tritan	Person who has tritanopia or tritanomaly.
Tritanomaly	Type of anomalous trichromatism in which there is reduced retinal sensitivity to blue light. An abnormally high amount of blue light is needed when mixing blue and green to match a given blue-green stimulus. Occurs in about 1 in a million people.
Tritanopia	Type of dichromatic colour vision deficiency in which blue and yellow are confused. There is a lack of retinal response

	to blue and yellow. Wavelengths longer than 570 nm are seen as red and those shorter than 570 nm are seen as green or bluish-green. Is more likely to be acquired than congenital, and can occur as a result of retinal disease, diabetes, glaucoma, retinitis pigmentosa etc. Congenital tritanopia is very rare and occurs in around five men and three women out of 100 000.
Tropicamide	An anticholinergic drug, used in the form of eye drops to dilate the pupil.
Tonus	A normal state of continuous slight tension in muscle tissue that facilitates its response to stimulation.
Uncompensated	Failure of the visual system to cope with heterophoria, uncompensated heterophoria.
Uncrossed disparity	Fixation disparity induced when the object is further from the eyes than the point of fixation and so is focused on the nasal retina.
Unilateral	Involving one side only.
V-pattern	Relative increase in exophoria on up gaze, or esophoria on down gaze.
Version	Movement of both eyes together.
Vision	Level of vision, usually measured using a vision testing chart, when the patient is not corrected.
Visual acuity	Level of vision, usually measured using a vision testing chart, when the patient is wearing their full correction.
Visual field	The area within which objects are visible to the immobile eye at any given time.
Visual field defect	Loss of retinal sensitivity (vision) in an area or areas of the visual field
Vitreous chamber	Space between the retina, the ciliary body and the post lenticular space of Berger, that is filled with vitreous humour
Vitreous humour	Clear, colourless, transparent jelly that fills the posterior segment of the (vitreous) eye.

Art of Clinical Practice in Optometry
AUTHOR BIOGRAPHIES

Frank was a professor in learning innovation and is currently a professor in clinical optometry with expertise in the fields of binocular vision, paediatric optometry, low vision, the effects of nutrition on long term eye health and quality assurance and enhancement in higher education. He is past-head of optometry at a leading UK optometry school where he was also lead clinician in the investigation and management of binocular vision anomalies. Prior to this he led a course on further investigative techniques. He was also an examiner for the College of Optometrists in binocular vision, further investigation and abnormal ocular conditions. He has co-investigated and co-managed hundreds of cases of binocular vision anomalies with orthoptists and ophthalmologists, lectured and led workshops in many countries and provided quality assurance expertise to optometry faculty in the UK, Ireland, Denmark, Pakistan and Singapore. He was part of an EU funded project where he assisted in the development of a low vision curriculum in Palestine and Jordan and another EU project where he developed online training material for carers working with older people with hearing and vision impairment. He has authored many research and clinical training articles and book chapters as well as five books. He is Co-Founder Director of the online professional development platform EyeTools.

Hannah is a Reader in Optometry at Aston University. Her educational experience has included teaching on undergraduate and postgraduate programmes for over 17 years, and she has developed expertise in the delivery of distance learning materials. She has recently been recognised as a Principal Fellow of Advance HE in the UK, is a reviewer for the UK National Teaching Fellowship programme and is also a member of Advance HE's Strategic Advisory Group on Diversity and Inclusion in higher education. Dr Bartlett graduated in 2000 with a First Class Honours in Optometry, and completed her PhD in Ocular Nutrition in 2005. She was appointed as Lecturer in Optometry in 2007 and has managed courses including Primary Ocular Examination, Low Vision and Paediatrics, Effective Communication and Retinal and Macular Disorders. In 2008 she was awarded an Aston Excellence Award for teaching. Her administrative responsibilities have included Careers Tutor, Admissions Tutor, International Tutor, First Year Tutor, and is currently appointed as Programme Director for the Optometry & Clinical Practice collaborative degree programme between Aston University and Parkway College of Nursing and Allied Health in Singapore. Her research has been disseminated in the form of around 50 peer-reviewed papers as well as four book chapters. In addition, her research has informed the education of peers in countries such as the US, Belgium, Singapore, South Africa, and Tanzania. Hannah's research portfolio is broadly based around the role of nutrition in ocular disease, but has included the development and evaluation of ophthalmic instrumentation, clinical trials, the development of hand-held technologies for people with low vision, and investigations of the psychology of nutritional behaviour. This range of research has been made possible through her collaborations with engineers, computer scientists, clinicians and health psychologists, and is linked by the aim to impact on the lives of those people living with ocular diseases.

Mark is a senior lecturer in Aston University's Optometry School and has taught visual biology, ophthalmic methods and research skills over the last 30 years. He has developed a suite of simulators for streak retinoscopy, subjective refraction, the cover test and for encouraging adoption of the problem orientated eye examination approach when making decisions about tentative diagnoses and referral urgency. These simulators draw upon current best practise and provide formative and summative feedback.

INDEX

A

AC/A ratio.......................... 161, 173, 174
Accommodative facility............... 161, 164
Accommodative insufficiency.............. 162
Amplitude of accommodation... 45, 46, 62, 73, 74
Amsler grid............................ 99, 134-136
Anisocoria 33, 215
Anomalous retinal correspondence....... 87
Anterior chamber... 93, 100, 151-158, 191, 202, 218
Applanation 104, 108, 215
ARC 87, 161, 168-172
Asthenopia 5

B

Bagolini lenses..................... 161, 170-172
Binocular addition........................... 69, 72
Binocular balancing.................. 69, 70, 72
Binocular indirect ophthalmoscopy..... 139, 141, 144
Brückner test............................. 1, 27, 28

C

Cardiff Acuity Cards 19
City University test 133
Colour vision 99, 132, 133, 223
Confrontation 121, 122
Cover test. 1, 29, 34, 35, 37-42, 51-56, 78, 83, 88, 161, 168, 170, 173, 178, 179

D

Diffuse illumination 97, 98, 192, 193
Dim-bright pupillary test 31
Diplopia 5, 6, 54, 56, 170, 217
Direct and consensual reflexes 30
Direct focal illumination 159
Direct ophthalmoscopy.............. 77, 93, 95
Duction............................ 51, 53, 54, 217

E

Eccentric fixation......................... 161, 175
Esoslip 92
Exoslip 92

F

Faculty of Ophthalmologists chart 20
Family medical history 2, 9
Family ocular history............................ 2, 9
Fixation disparity 87, 89-91, 164, 166, 168, 169, 220
Flashes and floaters 6
Fluorescein staining............. 183, 201, 202
Focimetry.. 1, 25
Fusional reserves 161, 180

G

General health.................................... 2, 8
Goldmann perimeter.................... 112, 113
Goldmann tonometer.......................... 104
Goniolens 151, 152, 153, 154, 156

H

Heterophoria...... 34-42, 78, 79, 83, 87, 91, 178, 179, 215-217, 219-221, 224
Heterotropia.... 34-42, 47, 78, 83, 168-173, 178, 179, 221
Hirschberg corneal reflexes............... 1, 29
History and symptoms 2, 10, 12, 13, 73
Humphrey visual field analyser..... 99, 117, 118

I

Indirect illumination.............................. 197
Institute of Optometry near card 22
Interpupillary distance............... 57, 58, 174
Ishihara test.. 132

J

Jump convergence 161, 177

K

Kay Pictures 18
Keeler Crowded/Uncrowded cards 17
Keratometer................................183-187
Kinetic perimetry........................ 111, 112

L

LH distance acuity symbols 18

Lid eversion 188, 206
LOFTSEA 3, 4, 5
LogMAR..16, 22
Low neutral dynamic retinoscopy.161, 163

M

Maclure chart bar reading book 21
Maddox rod............................... 77-79, 173
Maddox wing.................77, 79, 83-85, 173
Mallett Unit..........87, 89-92, 161, 168, 169
Monocular estimate method.................162
Motor fusion 180

N

Near addition 73, 111
Near fixation retinoscopy 65
Near point of convergence.............43, 166

O

Ocular history.......................................2, 7
Oculomotility 1, 41, 50, 55, 178

P

Pelli-Robson chart 137, 138
Perkins tonometer................................105
Pinhole test 23
Posterior segment.....77, 95, 144, 221, 224
Practical near acuity chart (PNAC) 23
Prism cover test 178
Pulsair..................................99, 101, 102
Pupil function 30

R

RAF rule........................... 43, 45, 46, 222
Reason for visit 2, 3
Retinoscopy 62, 65, 222

S

Sensory fusion 180
Simultaneous prism cover test 179
Slit-lamp direct ophthalmoscopy 147
Snellen 14-18, 21, 22, 35, 164-166
Soft contact lenses............................. 207
Specular reflection 200
Stereopsis 47-49
Subjective refraction..................... 67, 217
Supra-threshold tests 124
Swinging flash light test................. 30, 31

T

TNO... 47, 49
Tonometer.... 99, 101, 102, 104, 105, 107-109
Trial frame .. 14, 57, 59, 60, 62, 63, 68, 70, 74, 78, 81, 83, 86, 88, 168, 173, 221, 223

V

Vergence facility.......................... 161, 166
Visual field analysis............................ 110
Visuoscopy.. 175

W

Wratten 12 filter........................... 183, 204